Aurelio Bianchi, Anthony George Baker, Felix Regnault, M. Anastasiades

Translation of Lectures delivered by Aurelio Bianchi

On the Phonendoscope and its practical Application

Aurelio Bianchi, Anthony George Baker, Felix Regnault, M. Anastasiades

Translation of Lectures delivered by Aurelio Bianchi
On the Phonendoscope and its practical Application

ISBN/EAN: 9783337187385

Printed in Europe, USA, Canada, Australia, Japan

Cover: Foto ©ninafisch / pixelio.de

More available books at **www.hansebooks.com**

TRANSLATION OF LECTURES DELIVERED BY

AURELIO BIANCHI, M.D., - - - Parma.

Professor of Preparatory Clinical Medicine and of Pathology,

ON

THE PHONENDOSCOPE

AND

ITS PRACTICAL APPLICATION.

(Chapters I, II and III of this book are the English translation of lectures delivered by
Professor Aurelio Bianchi, and it is the direct intention of the publishers
that this book shall not be mistaken for the complete book
on Phonendoscopy in course of preparation.)

With Thirty-seven Illustrations.

WITH TRANSLATIONS OF SPECIAL ARTICLES BY

FELIX REGNAULT, M. D., ... France.

M. ANASTASIADES, M. D., ... Greece.

TRANSLATED BY

A. GEORGE BAKER, A. M. M. D.,

Physician in-Chief of the Chinese Medical Dispensary, Philadelphia, and author of
prize essays entitled " The Revival of Learning," and
" The Germans in America," Etc.

This book may be procured in Europe from
Martin Wallach, Nachfolger, Cassel, Germany.

PHILADELPHIA, U. S. A.

GEORGE P. PILLING & SON.

1898.

PREFACE.

The instrument which Professor Eugenio Bazzi and myself introduced at the International Medical Congress in Rome, in April, 1894, and to which we gave an absolutely new name —that of " Phonendoscope "—has quickly and permanently proven to be a substitute for the old Stethoscope, because it answered the purposes of the semiological examinations of to-day much better than it does.

It was, therefore, but natural that it should have found many warm friends, and that former opponents have since been converted to its use, and that a number of imitators and would-be improvers should have put in an appearance.

A work of this kind must necessarily speak of two subjects, the one referring to the past, and mentioning all those, who by changing the old Stethoscope, brought about the perfection and advance in the construction and effect of that instrument ; the other must refer to the present, speaking of those who have imitated our instrument and changed it.

The first part of the subject exhausts itself just here ; but the second can only be commenced later on, if any occasion should arise, and may be continued by ourselves.

I am not driven to this work by the thought of useless historical research or criticism, but by the necessity of setting right all features in their relations to each other to give each one his dues, which he deserves, in the accomplishment and use of the means of examining the sounds of the human organs, and to prevent others, who do not understand the scientific principles which are embodied in our apparatus, from getting the wrong impression, and from believing that it originated not by the thorough application and considerable study of many years, but that it owes its existence to a mere adoption of the researches of others.

To come to a clear understanding as to what our instrument ought to be, it took me nearly fifteen years of study and comparative examinations. Prof. Bazzi, who was willing to try and give my idea a practical form, was required to make many experiments and trials, and only after careful and patient study did we feel satisfied with our apparatus.

Prof. Bazzi in constructing the instrument put into it his profound knowledge of the physical laws, and I all the love and practical experience which I had acquired in this field, by the constant and faithful study of the human organs.

AURELIO BIANCHI, M. D.

TRANSLATOR'S PREFACE.

In making the following translations it has been my aim and object always to present the ideas of the various authors, as they were presented in the original productions.

Anyone familiar with one or more of the languages used on the Continent of Europe will appreciate the fact, when I say, that besides the languages in use among the ordinary people there is a so-called "University Tongue." This all professors think it their duty to use in their lectures and various literary productions. This "University Tongue" is somewhat confusing to the ordinary scholar, who may be able to read and speak the vernacular of the people. It seems to be the aim of all these professors to frame their sentences in a peculiar way, and with many circumlocutions, often covering a whole page or more by one single sentence. The ordinary reader is sure to forget the subject with which the sentence started by the time he gets to the end of it. We Americans do not express our thoughts after this fashion. Our sentences, even in works of a technical character, are mostly short and plain, so that he who reads may understand.

In the following pages I have tried to avoid these complications. I have tried, however, in every case, to give the exact idea and meaning of the author. I have also endeavored to render the ideas in an idiom which is easy to follow, and as nearly to our accepted standard as possible. Each language has its own peculiar idiom. In translating articles, therefore, which were written by authors belonging to different nationalities, the greatest care is required by the translator, so as not to fall into their way of constructing his sentences, but to remain true to "Uncle Sam's" pure American way of expressing himself. I leave it to the reader to judge how far I have succeeded in this my arduous undertaking. Hoping that all who read this little volume may derive the benefit which it is intended to convey, I remain,

Yours truly,

A. GEORGE BAKER, A. M. M. D.,
The Translator.

CONTENTS.

LIST OF ILLUSTRATIONS.

CHAPTER I.

THE PHONENDOSCOPE AND ITS PRACTICAL APPLICATION.

By Professor Aurelio Bianchi.

One of the principal endeavors of the learned men of the present century was directed towards the discovery of something which should carry to the ear of the examiner the sounds by which the internal processes and changes might be determined.

It may be asserted, with truth, that the whole basis of this principle of Semiotics, insofar as the same rests upon the different sounds which are produced in the organism, has been established within the present century. The knowledge of this all-important part of the medical science, in past centuries, was very imperfect and unreliable.

It was perceived that in order to make these sounds audible and distinct, instruments were needed. These sounds were too weak to be perceived without them. Therefore, the means by which these sounds might be carried to the ear of the observer were brought into requisition.

The first instrument of this kind was introduced by Laenneck, and was called the Stethoscope. It consisted of a wooden cylinder or tube, widened at each end, the smaller end of which was applied to the part of the body to be examined, whilst the ear of the examiner was applied to the other. It was called Stethoscope, because it was believed that the most important sounds were produced in the chest, which in Greek is called Stethos.

Further progress was made in Auscultation. Instead of the wooden cylinder other instruments of different material, of greater or lesser size were produced, but they were always called Stethoscope, and they were intended to carry the sounds directly to one ear of the examiner.

At the same time progress was made in the scientific knowledge of percussion, for the sounds produced by percussion show the nature of the interior, as modified by the different layers of muscles and skin, which modify the sound, according to the thickness or thinness of these outer walls.

In percussion an instrument was used which is named the percussion-hammer The hand, or the Pleximeter, were used to modify the sounds produced by the hammer. This instrument was sometimes round and flat, sometimes bi-convex, or elliptic, and was generally made of wood or ivory.

The sounds produced in this manner were only partially carried to the ear, because a good deal of the sound thus produced was lost in the surrounding atmosphere. Weak sounds, thus produced, could hardly be perceived.

An improved Stethoscope, one end of which was applied to the body, with two tubes, one for each ear, invented by the Americans, Drs. Camman and Clarke, was a marked advance, and the benefits derived from it were greater than those of the first instrument. The sounds produced by percussion were more accurately perceived.

The investigations made by myself by means of the Stethoscope, which consisted of two pieces of wood and two tubes, and then also by means of the Microphone, which produced sounds still more accurately, inspired me with the thought to search for an instrument which should not lose the minor sounds, as is the case with the Stethoscope; nor exaggerate them, as is the case, when the Microphone is used, and which should produce the natural sounds of the organism, as well as the artificial ones, which are produced by percussion, without changing the pitch of any and each particular sound.

An esteemed physicist, Prof. Eugene Bazzi, gave his consent, to give expression to this thought, which had originated in my mind, and was willing to make a number of practical experiments, and thus, an instrument or apparatus was produced which possessed all the desired qualities, not only for the purpose of making medical examinations and investigations, but also for the purpose of ascertaining the most minute sounds which are produced by living bodies of whatever sort, whether these sounds be natural or artificial.

This instrument was called Phonendoscope (*i. e.*, an instrument which carries to the outside sounds which originate within an organism); and thus it came to pass that my idea was put into practice, and a method of auscultation and percussion, the slightest effect of which is united with the greatest simplicity, and by means of the intelligence and patient labors of the thorough physicist, was fully realized.

The instruments made by the firm of Martin Wallach, Nachfolger, in Cassel (sold by their agents in America, Geo. P. Pilling & Son, Philadelphia), are the most perfect. It is about the size of a large watch, and consists of a metallic box with two vibrating plates, by means of which the instrument is placed upon the body to be examined. Two gum tubes serve as conductors of the sound from the body to the ears. In many cases, and for some purposes, one tube alone suffices, but the other must also be attached to the instrument. By means of a small buttoned rod, which, when needed, may be secured to the lower vibrating plate, makes it possible to localize the point to be examined by auscultation, i. e. the point to be examined, with the instrument, by the ear. In this way you are enabled to perceive the sound-waves, even at a distance from the vibrating body, with very little loss of sound, and without change of rhythm or intensity, and this vibration is perceived with single or double sensibility, according to the wish of the examiner.

The Phonendoscope does not produce any material change in the observation of the vibrations of the body examined, but carries the sound waves, without change or dispersion to the ears, and delivers them as a whole; as, for instance, murmurs, or noises, just as they exist in the locality of the body which is being examined, in their absolute perfection, and makes it possible for us to perceive the same, with either simple or double strength and sensibility, as we may be inclined to use either one or both tubes, which carry the sound to the ears.

All objections which might be advanced as regards the exaggeration of sound, or changes of the same, or abnormal sensitiveness, etc., are vain; on the contrary, the Phonendoscope surpasses all other instruments of the kind, on account of the small volume, as well as by its peculiar adaptability for the purpose of examining any and all sounds produced in the body to be examined. No other instrument, made heretofore, can be compared to this, which surpasses all others in accuracy and usefulness.

The practical application of the Phonendoscope is not difficult. If it is intended to serve for the auscultation of the internal parts of the body, we simply lay the instrument upon the part to be examined, and press it down a little, and according to the sensibility and effect we desire to produce, we simply place one or both tubes into the ear or ears. But if the examination is to be made upon a single part, and upon a circumscribed area, then all that is required is to screw the little buttoned rod into the lower plate, and press more or less strongly upon the external part or point. Ultimately, if the Phonendoscope is to be applied for the artificially produced conditions, which may be induced at will, then the buttoned rod must always be used. In most of these cases one tube alone suffices for auscultation.

The sounds produced by the percussion hammer on the Pleximeter, or with the finger upon the finger, are, under the circumstances, too strong for the Phonendoscope. A gentle rubbing upon the surface of the body is quite sufficient. A simple rubbing with the index finger about the point to be examined. One rule only must be followed in order to become proficient in the application of the Phonendoscope. When you apply the instrument see to it that the body and the tubes do not touch anything, and do not rub against any article of dress, nor against each other, for such rubbing produces sound, which does not belong to the area to be examined. This precaution is easily taken.

The practical auscultation by means of the Phonendoscope, so that the different sounds and noises in the body may be distinctly observed, is easily and quickly accomplished. The ordinary knowledge furnished us by Semiotics, in regard to the different noises, is sufficient. But, on the other hand, great care is required, in auscultation with the Phonendoscope, when we produce artificial sounds in the body. It requires some study, although, some rules have been obtained in Semiotics, according to which we must measure the sounds and noises.

These rules, when applied, modulate sound, and present it in a higher or lower pitch ; this requires special care and attention.

Several gum tubes, more or less, as may be desired, may be attached to the Phonendoscope ; and thus, a larger or smaller number of persons may listen simultaneously, and the lecturer may speak on the semiological value of a particular sound, which may be observed by all who listen to it at once.

Considered from this standpoint the Phonendoscope offers every guarantee for the correctness of the results of an examination, inasmuch as several experts may convince themselves of the existing condition, at one and the same time. For clinical instruction this instrument enables the teacher to explain the value and character of the sounds to a number of his hearers, who may listen, with him, while he analyzes them. To a certain extent, the sounds may be weakened, when so many listen at once ; but, nevertheless, the sounds artificially called forth, or naturally produced, may be analyzed with certainty, inasmuch as six or eight persons may take part in the examination, all of whom observe the same sound, at the same time, and thus come to a definite conclusion, in regard to the sounds which they hear. If there is a difference this will only depend on the difference in the organs of hearing of the different observers.

After thus enumerating the main characteristics of Phonendoscopical examinations we now come to its practical application in the practice of medicine.

Its uses in midwifery and gynæcology, as well as in surgery, offer themselves as objects of study to us, at this time, in this branch of the science, and it appears necessary to me to make my investigations, with a view to point to, and apply the Phonendoscope in semiology, more especially to the internal parts, in relation to practical treatment.

If you place the Phonendoscope with one of its vibrating plates upon a living body, or if a living body rests upon it wholly or in part, whilst the tubes are in the ears of the examiner, he will notice a rhythmical sound, of greater or lesser intensity, and equality, which is continued as long as the instrument is in contact with the living body.

This noise, which originates in the vascular system, and in the muscular walls, is of different intensity, as is self-evident, and is in close relation with the circulation of the blood, and the blood pressure, more or less ; and, on the other hand, also results from the condition of the muscles, at the point of investigation.

This noise was called Dermatophony, and could only be proved thus far, with the very sensible Microphone, which, owing to the peculiar construction of the parts, was not easily transportable.

If you place the Phonendoscope over a joint, or on the ending of a muscle, and then make a movement of the joint or muscle, or if you pass a steady (constant) or an inductive current through them, then the exaltations or actions, in all their variations and distinctions are perceived by the Phonendoscope, and the instrument, in this way, reveals the normal or abnormal condition of the parts examined. The same is true of a bone that may be broken, or which is believed to have been broken. If you place the instrument upon that part, then if there is a fracture, the least movement of the fractured parts will reveal the grating noise of the fractured bones, which will be distinctly audible. The injured man does not suffer any pain, from this procedure.

The auscultation of the tones of the sounds and noises that are caused by the exaltation of the respiration is easily accomplished, and distinctly perceived, with the Phonendoscope. This is done by placing one plate of the instrument upon the breast, and by pressing it gently against the chest-wall. The surface of about six inches is thus examined, and the condition of the lungs, may, by examination, be revealed, in a very short time.

In order to examine the sounds accurately in different parts, upon which the plate of the Phonendoscope cannot be laid, all that is necessary is to touch the parts with the little buttoned rod. By means of this rod the given tones of the lungs can be ausculted, whether it be the apexes, or partitions on the sides. This may be done by listening with one or both ears, according as it may appear best, and according to the sounds produced inside, whether they be stronger or weaker. Thus respiration in all its peculiarities may be accurately analyzed. The least abnormal phenomena, which show themselves, will be perceived. Just on this very account the Phonendoscope possesses an undisputed superiority over all other means employed for auscultation.

When we auscult the larynx or trachea we hear clearly the acoustic manifestations, which, by the passage of the air through these organs, are called into existence, and the locality may be accurately pointed out, where modifications caused by roughness, sthenosis, etc., exist.

We now pass on to the auscultation of the acoustic manifestations of the circulation of the blood, and the sounds produced by the blood-wave, and those which are heard in the larger blood vessels, and also those which originate in the heart ; *i e.*, noises which can be distinguished from each other by their peculiarities. This kind of auscultation may be accomplished either with the plate, or with the little rod ; this last especially, for the purpose of those tones, *i. e.*, those points, where the heart sounds are most clearly and distinctly perceived, or heard.

Not only the points of the strongest intensity of sounds, which are produced by the valves of the heart, but also the diffusive sounds may be fixed, as well as the point where these sounds, produced by this central cause, have their stopping place, or where the sounds of another neighboring central point become more distinctly audible. In this way then, we are enabled, with the greatest facility, to make a diagnosis of the condition of the heart and its action in general, and the peculiar action and condition of its parts in particular.

Here you will permit me to make a few observations on the new art now made possible of examining with the Phonendoscope, namely, about comparative auscultation.

This examination is rather more of a clinical than practical nature, not only for the purpose of instruction in the classroom, but for its manifold usefulness in the actual practice of the physician.

For the purpose of comparative auscultation two instruments are requisite, which must be placed on the two different points which are to be examined and compared. One tube of each instrument must be placed in the ears. In this way we accomplish the conveying of the sounds of the two points which are to be examined at once, in order that the sounds produced in each may be compared with each other, and the sound-wave is to be interrupted by taking now one and then the other tube into the ear and out of it, or the tubes may be compressed alternately, and the sound stopped now in one and then in the other. In this way the sounds and noises of the different points may be differentiated and compared most accurately.

In this way, too, may be heard at one and the same time, the workings of both lungs, in one and the same individual, or those of certain different parts, in the lungs of the patient, and the corresponding part of one who is perfectly well, and in his normal condition.

The same comparative auscultation may be instituted on the heart of two individuals, a sick man, and one who is well. Heretofore this new method of investigation has not been possible for want of a suitable instrument, but now, this can be easily accomplished without any trouble. This new method may be applied to many other parts.

To come back to the use of the Phonendoscope in simple auscultation, we may see its usefulness in the examination of the lower parts of the abdomen, which heretofore has been but seldom or not at all applied to these parts. The question here is not as to the murmuring noises only, as is the case when we examine the heart and lungs, but also the noises which we hear when we examine the stomach and the liver, and, in some cases, in superfluous meteorism, or by too much liquid being deposited or lodged in the lower parts of the abdomen, but also those sounds which are of a local character, and which are caused by pathological or physiological conditions. All acoustic manifestations which originate in the stomach and intestines, as likewise the process of digestion, which is going on in these organs, may be observed by the physician, by means of this instrument.

This is an entirely new semiotic, which by study and practice offers many advantages. But the variation of sounds which we perceive by this method of examination is truly astonishing. You may notice the absolute silence that is but seldom interrupted in cases of inactivity and paralysis of the muscular coating of the stomach and intestinal tube. You may hear a noise, as if grating or grinding to and fro, of different strength, according to the rapidity with which the contents of these organs are moving onward. Much depends upon the nature of these contents, whether they be of a gasey or of a liquid character, and whether they are mixing under the muscular process of the intestines ; thus, you hear the gurgling sound in the bowels, when the existing gas escapes from a narrow into a wider passage, through liquid substance, and moves either forward or backward, or up and down. You hear the dull, but at the same time rhythmical sound caused by the exertions which are used by the stomach as it discharges its contents through the pyloric orifice into the duodenum.

In some cases of tuberculosis of the omentum or peritonium, or of peritonitis, when the dry rubbing sounds of the surfaces against each other are distinctly audible, whilst the sounds produced by hydatic cysts, as those produced by the peristaltic movements of the mucous membrane of the bowels, are distinctly perceptible.

I will not speak of the Phonendoscopic auscultation of the brain, in order that I may have more time to explain the artificially produced exaltation of the organs, which are to be examined with the Phonendoscope. In this way we are enabled to give accurately the form, the location, and the relations of those organs, whilst this method of examination enables us to find out their tonicity and density.

By this examination the little rod of the Phonendoscope is applied to a point, which has been made bare by the removal of all clothing, and which is pressed firmly upon the skin, whilst, for the most part, the use of one ear tube suffices. It is sufficient if you rub with the index finger over the surface in the neighborhood of the little rod, which will produce some little vibration in the parts, which may be distinctly heard, which differs, however, according to the density and tonicity of the organ which is being examined. After this you rub in the same manner, at some little distance from the first spot. If you can produce no sound or but little, then you continue to rub toward the button of the little rod, and with a pencil mark the place, where the vibration takes place, and is similar to the vibration excited in the region of the buttoned rod. If you continue to make a circular motion about the rod, by carefully rubbing from circumference towards the central point, and in doubtful cases, from the little rod towards the outer circle, then you will be enabled to fix a number of points, which will reveal the condition of the internal organs, within this certain radius that has been examined.

A few rules are to be observed, and are easily understood and followed.

It is better to let the buttoned rod rest upon the soft parts, and not upon any bone, because in the latter case, the vibrations or sounds of the organs will be similar to that which is heard in the bone, and thus might be mistaken, and greater care is required to differentiate where the vibration or sound of each organ stops, or where that which originates in the bone does not continue to go on.

It is further to be observed that by too much pressure, with the buttoned rod upon the surface, the sound or vibration produced there may suppress that of the internal organs, and even the vibration of the skin itself will be partially weakened by too much pressure. This possible cause for error must therefore be avoided.

It is necessary that the buttoned rod shall rest upon one part of the internal organ which is not covered by any other organ, otherwise it will be impossible to fix the point within the circumference, with any degree of accuracy. For example, when the heart is being examined, with the Phonendoscope, then the rod must be placed over the heart, where the heart is free, and not overlapped by the tips of the lungs, but in the mediastinum, or place where the heart lies nearest to the chest-wall. When we examine the stomach, then, only those parts are to be chosen, which are not covered by the left tip of the liver.

It is also necessary to place the little rod over various selected points of different organs, in order to ascertain the size and place of these organs. For example, for the examination of the heart the little rod must be placed within the fourth intercostal space near the sternum, and for the liver in the seventh intercostal space upon the nipple of the right breast;

for the stomach likewise in the seventh intercostal space, but placed on the left nipple.

If an organ happens to be very much enlarged, then the rod must be placed over it in several points successively. As *e. g.* for the liver first in the seventh intercostal space on the right nipple, then in the ninth under the axilla, and in the sword-like continuation of the twelfth joint of the spinal column.

For the stomach, the rod is first placed in the seventh intercostal space upon the left nipple, then on the linia alba near the curve of the short ribs.

If an organ is divided into several parts of segments, like the lungs, divided by a middle wall, and space for the heart, or is separated by ligaments, like the hepatic bands, or if an organ contains substances of different consistency, as the stomach, containing both gas and food, then the little rod must be placed at different points successively, because these organs, as a whole, are divided into parts, which are separated by spaces, ligaments and substances of different thicknesses, which hinder the sounds from passing through the whole organ at once, and at the same time.

If we proceed in this way, and by the method marked out above, then, truly, the results are most convincing and astonishing. There are certain points which may be fixed in a given locality; the parts of the lungs in their two sides; the Nivean of the liquid contents of the pleura and abdominal cavity, the contour and outline of the stomach, together with the shifting of the contents, according to the position in which the patient may happen to lie; so with the chambers of the heart, and the flaps or lobes of the liver, etc, etc.

If any organ is to be examined which is covered by some other, but elastic organ, which weakens the sounds, then the rubbing with the finger over the skin must be conducted with more force. For example:—in case of an emphysematous lung, which may overlap the heart we must rub with more force, than would be required in that locality, where the heart lies in more direct contact with the chest-wall.

By means of this method of investigation we are enabled to draw the size of the organ upon the skin, as accurately as if

we could place their shadow there, with this exception, that
the shadow forms a visible spot, whereas, in this way, the pho-
nentical shadow may be drawn whole, and in all its parts and
subdivisions, into which these organs may happen to be divided,
by walls and furrows.

These results had already been obtained with the double
Stethoscope; and my observations made since 1882, which I have
published, are confirming them.   But by means of the Phonendoscope we can examine with greater accuracy, and far less
trouble, and without loss of time.

(The speaker here referred to the successful examinations,
each by itself, of the different organs, as the lungs, heart,
stomach, liver, duodenum, bladder, spleen, kidneys, and especially referred to Prof. A. Bianchi's intention to give further instruction in the future, on the use of the Phonendoscope).

As you see, the plans and drawings mark out the size of
the organs most accurately.   The plans and drawings of the
different organs may be made without loss of time.   They
mark the location of each organ, and their relations one to
another.   Thus we may observe how far the lobes of the lung
overlap the heart.   You may observe how far the liver elevates
the diaphragm and the degree or extent to which the pyloris is
covered by the liver.   We may fix the extent of the cardia of
the stomach, and you can study the curves of the colon and of
the stomach as well.

Not only this: We may study displacements and changes
in the structure, and, by means of this method, we may outline,
by drawings, these very changes, and thus place them in reality
before our very eyes.

For this purpose the organs are first drawn, whilst the
patient is lying on his back, then he is to get up quickly, and
stand upon his feet; or he may be first ordered to lie on his
right, then on his left side, and thus we are enabled to fix with
certainty, the location of the different organs, in the different
positions of the patient.

Finally, even the shifting of the organs, from place to
place, may also be observed, as caused by the different functions
which they perform; thus for example, whilst we cause the
patient to take a deep inspiration, we may not only observe how

far his lungs expand, but also what motions they impart to other neighboring organs.

These few short examples show how far the use of the Phonendoscope may be carried in medical practice. Many examinations which heretofore were most difficult to make, and those which could only be made in part, and very imperfectly, can now, by the aid of this instrument, be made with the greatest certainty and facility.

(The experiments which were made during the lecture in the presence of many physicians, were absolutely satisfactory, and Professors Rossoni, Queirolo, and Felice, confirmed the usefulness, and the advantages which they had derived from the use of the Phonendoscope, in their clinical examinations.

CHAPTER II.

PHONENDOSCOPY OF THE ORGANS, ESPECIALLY CONCERNING THE STOMACH AND ITS CONTENTS, WITH EXPERIMENTS.

The method of examining with the Phonendoscope, or, as it is now called, "Phonendoscopy," differs as much from the ordinary method of auscultation and percussion, as differ the various other instruments that are used for that purpose from the Phonendoscope. By this method the vibrations which originate in the organism, while performing its various functions, or those which are called into existence by external influences, are carried directly, and without dispersion or change, to the ear of the examiner. And it is on this account that I make the positive assertion, that the Phonendoscope is superior to all other instruments in use at the present day. It alone reveals the exact condition of things as they exist in the organism. Neither the Stethoscope nor the old percussion method could make audible sounds with anything like the same degree of accuracy. I have repeatedly referred to its value and uses, when employed in exploring the internal parts, since my first invention and use of the instrument in 1894.

(1) At that time I used an ordinary Stethoscope to which I attached more rubber tubes, with olives for the ears. I also devised another Stethoscope, in the form of a little bell, to which I fastened the tubes directly. (2) This instrument had enabled me to obtain important results, but it does not possess the accuracy and importance of the Phonendoscope. It is only since I had this perfect instrument that I could get absolutely new results, and could state, with the greatest accuracy, the most minute modifications in the formation of the various organs.

---

(1) Dell auscultazione stetoscopica della percussione, kirista clinica, Bologna & Gaz. ospedali, Milano, 1881. Riforma medica, Napoli, 1885.
(2) Italian edition of the "Semiologie," by Eichhorst, vol. 1, 1885.

Bedersky in Kiew, (3) and Aufrecht in Magdeburg, have one after the other tried to use an instrument in the form of a bell similar to the one described by me since 1884, but the results obtained by them were not any better than mine, by the same identical instrument. The fact is that the Stethoscopes of Bedersky and Aufrecht have air chambers which are too large, and the vibrations become dispersed instead of concentrated. They are without the vibrating plate, and, therefore, cannot be used on an extensive surface with the same ease as on a surface of limited extent. Their instruments enable us to examine but a limited surface, and cannot be altered so as to meet the requirements of the examination.

Charles Verdin, of Paris, has expressed the opinion (4) after an accurate study of the Phonendoscope, that before this no similar instrument was in existence, and that all others which were produced in imitation of the same could not give the same results as the Phonendoscope, except those instruments which were correct copies of the original.

In a critical study (5) of the question concerning this subject I have tried to point out this fact most clearly, in the history of the instrument.

The commission nominated, with this end in view, by the "Societe' de Medicine" at Paris, (6) fully recognized the novelty and priority of the instrument, as well as the novelty of the method.

I.

The results which can be obtained by an examination with the Phonendoscope are very many, but they can be divided into two main sections :—

First :—They enable us to hear the sounds produced by the functions of the organs.

Second—They enable us also to hear the sounds which are produced artificially. As every sound is caused by vibration,

(3) Academie de Medicine, Paris, 1896.

(4) Aertze-Verein, Berlin, 1897

(5) Die Vorlanfer, Nachahamer & Abanderer des Phoneudoscops, Cassel, 1897.

(6) Lectures of the Societe de Medicine, Paris, March, 1896.

it is certain, that with the Phonendoscope, we can make audible the vibrations of bodies in general, and of the human body in particular, *i. e.*, those sounds which are caused by the normal or pathological functions of the body, as well as those vibrations which are caused artificially, in the organism, by any external means. For this reason it is sufficient, for instance, to pass the finger, with gentle pressure, over the surface of the body, or to observe the vibrations transmitted from a vibrating object, such as a tuning fork or vibrating rod.

I will not speak to you at this time about the first part which covers almost the entire field of auscultation. With the Phonendoscope you receive better and more accurate results, but the laws of this method do not differ from those of the ordinary auscultation.

Here I wish to remark that the doubts expressed by some (Egger and Grote) in regard to the modifications, the alterations and the deformity noticed in the sounds obtained by means of the Phonendoscope are without foundation. In these cases we have always to do with investigations and experiments, the technicality of the instrument not having been understood well enough, or with the faulty application of the instrument itself to the parts examined.

To obtain perfect results it requires rather strong pressure, with the lower surface of the Phonendoscope, or the little rod attached to it, according as we desire to examine a large, or a limited surface, otherwise the vibrations will become modified, and imperfect, and weakened, while passing through the different layers of varying thickness, *i. e.* muscles, skin, fatty tissue, bones, etc.

With a gradually increasing, rather strong pressure, we bring the different layers close to each other, and in this way we produce an almost even and dense mass. By means of this procedure the vibrations are well conducted through the artificially produced layer, and suffer only slight modifications and weakenings.

With this end in view we can make an experiment, as a limited auscultation of the sounds of the heart, at the point of this organ. When the Phonendoscope is simply placed upon the skin you will hear almost nothing, especially when the sounds are weak, and the tissues, lying above it, are very thick. By using pressure, you will hear better the more you increase it, but only up to a certain point, and then it will be the reverse; for too much pressure will, eventually, to a certain extent, smother the vibrations of the organ which is being examined.

II.

The most important and useful application of the Phonendoscope consists in making the artificially produced sounds audible for the purpose of ascertaining the formation and outline of the different parts of the body. The possibility of outlining the organs by auscultation in connection with percussion was mentioned by many of the older physicians and among these were Piorry and Laenneck. A practical application was made in 1841 by the two Americans, Cammau and Clarke. Their method of examining simply consisted in collecting the vibrations produced by a double stick of wood, and by another physician who used percussion. But this method was not of any practical importance because two physicians were required when it was applied, the one to auscult and the other to percuss; later on this method was partly employed by Barthey, Roger, Frederick McBride, Ewald and others, and for the reason mentioned, in but isolated cases.

In 1880 I again took up this method of examining with a double Stethoscope and made close observations and investigations, and found, after many trials and experiments, the laws by which I could apply it, as a real semiologic method, which may be applied in all cases of examinations of any part of the body, and to which I gave the name of "Stethoscopy," or the science of making audible the sounds produced by percussion. But the inconvenience of requiring an assistant to hold the instrument in its place was still there, while the other physician made the percussion, and auscultation. The writings produced in the line of these studies are rather lengthy, and I think it advisable to quote largely for the convenience of those who, perhaps, would like to make some experiments of this kind.

I continued my examinations by this method, and, in the meantime, I hunted for an instrument which should allow the physician to auscult at the same time while he himself produced the vibrations of the organs.

In 1894 I gained the conviction, with the help of Dr. Bazzi, Professor of Physic in Florence, that I had found the right method. By a great number of experiments we tried to make the instrument practical and suitable for all cases that might occur, and finally we produced such a one, and named it the "Phonendoscope" (ascertainer of the sounds in the interior parts of the body). This was in 1894, at the time when the Eleventh International Medical Congress met at Rome, in Italy.

The Phonendoscope made by Martin Wallach, Successor, in Cassel, Charles Verdin, in Paris, and George P. Pilling & Son, Philadelphia, U. S. A. was the most perfect, and other imitations and modifications which have appeared since were always inferior to the original instrument. The results of which we have spoken were obtained only by using the Phonendoscope made by the above-mentioned firms, and no other.

This period really marks the commencement of the study of the different parts of the body by means of artificially produced vibrations. In fact, in the Phonendoscope we have an instrument which makes it possible for us to examine the most minute point, or any part of the body, or limited area, and also the advantage, that by means of it every physician can practice auscultation with the greatest of ease, while he himself may produce artificial vibrations in the part which he examines. It is safe to say that this method has its real origin in the invention of the instrument, and for this reason I named it the "Phonendoscope."

III.

The phonendoscopy of the vibrations which we may wish to produce artificially is very simple. If you see it once applied you will be able to follow this method perfectly, without any trouble. All you require is a little application and the necessary practice. It has many advantages over the ordinary method of percussion, as it does not require lengthy experiments and but little practice. The experts in percussion are very few and scarce, but this method not only recommends itself for its facility of learning it but also for the simplicity of the means employed. It is sufficient to pass the point of the finger with gentle pressure along the line over the edge of the organ to be examined, to produce the vibrations necessary for the examination. In this way the physician does not become fatigued from percussion, and the persons nearby, who are otherwise engaged, are not disturbed by the sounds, and the individual under examination does not feel any disagreeable or painful sensation. Those who imagine that this method has the same limits as the ordinary percussion method are simply mistaken; for there are certain well-marked differences between both methods.

With the ordinary percussion method you cannot distinguish the separation which marks the lobes of the lungs, nor those of the heart, neither the two of the liver, nor can you distinguish the changes of the contents of the stomach, nor the cardiac or piloric end, sometimes not even the lower curve of the stomach, nor the posterior part of the spleen; also very often not the kidneys, nor the organs that are found in a liquid state, neither can you find the limits of the bones and the ends of the muscles, nor the fractures of bones. In one word, the results of phonendoscopy differ so much from those of the ordinary percussion method, that nobody would compare the one with the other. This proves that phonendoscopy is the scientific method of examining the form, extention, position, the changes and the respective relations of the parts of the body, which is founded upon the observation of sounds with the ear, made possible by the use of the Phonendoscope. The sounds observed are those which are produced by the vibrations, as much as possible, directly transmitted to the organ of a body we examine, being itself in vibrating motion, or of one producing such.

You can see what a large field for investigation has thus been opened by the Phonendoscope, and so various in its use and applications, in the different departments of medicine and the natural sciences. Through the co-operation of scientific thinkers and workers the highest results will be obtained by this method which it is possible to attain.

IV.

The theory is very simple. The body in which the vibrations are produced must transmit the same to the ear directly, more or less in their totality. To obtain these results three stages are necessary in the examinations:

First—That of producing vibrations,
Second—Transmitting the vibrations,
Third—That of noticing the vibrations.

(1) That stage producing of vibrations is caused by simply passing over the part or parts with the tip of the finger. The finger must be well pressed upon the part lying over the organ, and it is necessary to produce in the different layers the same degree of density, whether these layers be in direct or indirect contact with the different points of the organ to be examined or not. Therefore, the pressure, and passing over of the finger tips, will have to be stronger for the organs in the chest, than for those in the abdomen; and stronger for those parts covered by the organs of little density and little tension, than for those covered by very dense and well stretched organs; and stronger for the parts lying far beneath the surface of the body, than for those lying directly under it.

If the finger is not well pressed down the vibration will be a surface vibration, which may act by completely disturbing, and induce a series of fractional sounds and echoes, in the layers of different density, and this may hinder us from getting at all to the part which is to be examined. Here we must try and avoid the mistakes which have led to negative results in the examinations of different investigators, as Bouveret, Egger, Grote and a few others. In such a case one of these gentlemen would describe the lines of the skin, and not the projection or part of the organ which he tried to investigate by his examination.

(2) When the vibration is transmitted to the organ it will vibrate according to its density and tension. The vibrations of the organ will transmit themselves to the organs surrounding it and will undergo a series of reflexions and breaks, while passing through the intervening layers. To collect these vibrations it is necessary that the little stem or rod of the Phonen-

doscope be used, in order to produce an artificial continuity in
the density of the tissue, lying between the organ and the
Phonendoscope, and be made to vibrate ; and thus, the little
stem itself must be pressed upon the tissue of the organ which
is to be examined. Consequently, the little stem must be well
pressed against the wall of the body, and must be placed upon
the point which is in direct contact with the organ which is to
be examined. By not paying attention to these simple rules
the results will be negative. It is understood that we can only
approximate fixed points of observation. It is therefore necessary that we make out, first the organs lying near the surface,
and then the organs lying lower down, and then by putting the
little stem or rod on the space which is left free. In this way
I now would like to describe, first the lower limits of the right
lung, before describing the liver ; and the limits of the left
lung, before the spleen ; and the inner edge of the lungs, before
we look for the heart ; the lower edge of the liver, before marking the stomach, or the right kidney, or the colon on the right
side ; the lower edge of the stomach and the spleen, before the
colon on the left ; those of the spleen behind, before marking
the left kidney. In this way the topography of the intestines
will become very simple, and it will be sufficient to remember
the most elementary anatomical knowledge, in order to make
an exact outline of the various parts of the body.

(3) Noticing of the vibrations which are produced is in
itself very simple. If you put the little stem on the vibrating
body the vibrations transmitted by the little stem to the vibrating plate of the Phonendoscope will become condensed in its
little air chamber, and by means of the two tubes reaches the
outer ear at the tympanum which will thus be caused to vibrate.
We have, therefore, according to the physical laws which govern this department of science, the sensation of a more or less
powerful noise. This proves the fact that when the little stem
is in contact with any part of the body it conducts all the vibrations to the ear, which are produced upon the surface of the
body, and which correspond to that part of the body which is
being examined. If the vibrations are caused in the skin or
outer limits of a part of the body, then they are not at all, or
but very slightly, perceived. It is necessary to mark the point

with a pencil where the vibration ceases or diminishes. In
comparing all the parts obtained in this way, in one line, we
will get a figure which represents an outline of that part of the
body. This outline may be traced on the even walls of the
body (front or back, as the case requires), and almost of the
same size as the organ. On the sides however this outline will
be larger. These, then, are the laws which govern the shadow
to be observed, and one and the same part will give different
figures upon the wall of the body, according to the position
assumed by the patient. In this way the conical-shaped heart
will furnish an outline more like a round or triangular figure,
according as to whether it is more or less vertical to the wall
of the chest.

V.

The importance of this really extraordinary result received
by such simple means is confirmed in the post-mortem examinations (Schwalbe, Roux), and by experiments made upon
animals, and especially by means of the radioscope, which also
brings to light the changes taking place in the different organs.
If, for instance, you make an examination of the lower edge of
a lobe of the lungs, and cause the patient to exhale and inhale,
while passing over the part your finger in the proper manner,
you will see the line previously marked upon the skin displac-
ing itself, and moving either up or down, although the little
stem remains in the same place, and by this pressure the
displacement of the skin is prevented. You also see this when
tracing the outline of the empty stomach, and while allowing
the little stem to rest upon the same spot. But fill it with
liquid and all the edges of the neighboring organs will displace
themselves. The most clear and simplest experiment is the
following : You mark, in a standing position, the upper edge
of the liquid contents of the stomach, and, while leaving the
little stem in its position, raise with the hand the lower part of
the stomach. You continue at the same time to pass the finger
in a parallel line over the nivean of the liquid, and you find
that this displaces itself upward, according to the pressure
brought to bear against it at the lower part. In relieving the
pressure the nivean of the liquid will go down and take its
former position.

When we witness such a simple and clear experiment we cannot doubt the results of the method, and, I repeat it, that the isolated negative results are simply to be attributed to the insufficient knowledge of the common laws and their partial application in our method.

VI.

The outlines of the diagram of organs marked in such a way give us figures, very different from those which have become traditional in the manuels of semiology. For this very reason either the one or the other finds fault with the Phonendoscope for giving us an ideal and not the real figure of the organ. But this finding fault is most unjust. The ordinary percussion gives us the outlines of the organs very differently, because it is almost always performed while the individual is lying down, and, therefore, the organs are drawn into different positions, and are displaced backwards. The outline made in this way cannot be the same as the one received with the Phonendoscope, which is generally made while the individual is standing. And furthermore, in practicing phonendoscopy on a person lying down it will give more perfect results than the ordinary method of percussion. We are used to seeing in the manuels of semiology, as a rule, the organs drawn in the ordinary position, and in their mutual relations, as they are shown in the manuels of anatomy. But the form, position and mutual relations, as they are represented after death, are not the same as during the life, whether it be in a physiological view, or during a change produced by disease. The drawings made by means of the Phonendoscope, by the outlining of the organs on the wall of the body, as it were, by the shadow of the organ, the harmony of the phonendoscopic diagrams with those received by the X-rays (7) is the clearest proof of the correctness of this assertion.

VII.

The application of the method in medicine and in the sciences related to it are very numerous. Besides the physiological and pathological studies about the lungs, heart, liver, spleen, colon and kidneys, we have a large quantity of altogether new productions, in studies about the diseased products,

---

(7) Congress fur innere Medicine, Berlin, 1897.

transfilitration, new formations and about the changes caused by them in the various organs.

Here I will try to give the exact indications for the study of the stomach, the changes of its volume, the form, the position and the relations between the whole and its contents. The stomach cannot be considered as being like any other organ. It has thin walls, and can only be studied by means of its contents. If the stomach contains nothing but gases or liquid material, then it acts just the same as any other organ ; but if it contains liquids and gases it must be looked upon as composed of a gas chamber and liquid chamber of different density and tension. The total outline will therefore be obtained by the phonendoscopy of the gas chamber and of the liquid chamber. We therefore require two points of observation. We must first set the little stem upon the liquid chamber and then upon the gas chamber. These are like two separated organs, which are to be marked upon the skin by diagrams, one after the other, and which give the entire outline of the stomach, by uniting them both into a single diagram.

In my lectures to the class (8) I have demonstrated already that it is necessary to draw, first the lower edge of the liver, and that in putting the little rod below that line, on the left hemiclavicular line, we can find the outline of the stomach. This is the ordinary rule, but there are also exceptions, and it is well to know them in order to avoid any mistakes.

After taking food, when the liver is thick and sinks down to the left, and if the stomach contains much liquid, it is impossible to find the gas chamber, which is then entirely covered by the liver. Also if the spleen or the kidneys are enlarged, and the stomach is almost entirely covered by these organs. But if the stomach is pressed down by pressure from above, or is pushed away by a dense mass which is stronger than its walls, then the gas and liquid chambers are fully uncovered and are always easily traced, even though a person suffer with ascitis. In this way you can keep the drawings, and the relations of the stomach to the other neighboring organs, by photography or chromography and perceive from them the

---

(8) The three main forms of the stomach, the gastric curve within twenty-four hours. The difference in the digestion of liquids. (22-23½ 97.)

displacements by the process of digestion, and from many other causes. It is most interesting to follow in this way for several hours the displacement of the organ and the changes of its contents, and to be able to observe the action of the different foods and medicaments, by the comparison of the different drawings. In this way I have been able to draw the first complete gastric curve within twenty-four hours, and this drawing, the first one made, until now, I have deposited in the physiological laboratory of the University of Moscow.

Before finishing I wish to call your attention again to the importance and simplicity of the method.

With one single instrument, the Phonendoscope, and a pencil, with the aid of the point of the finger, and without the least inconvenience to the individual under examination, you can draw all parts of the body in a short time.

For this reason, phonendoscopy, during the last three years of its existence, has come into quite extensive use, and will slowly extend itself more and more, and certainly the time is not far distant when it will be mentioned in all the manuels of semiology, besides the simple methods of percussion and auscultation.

A new method, in order to make its way through the world, must first become known and gather support. It must become known to the hospital physicians, as well as the private practitioners, and must be supported by the investigators who are the real friends of scientific truth and discoveries.

The examinations following this lecture were witnessed, each time, by five physicians at once, and which resulted in quickly and easily fixing the lungs, the heart, the liver, the stomach, the spleen, and their outlines, making apparent the displacements of the lungs during inhalation and exhalation, the shifting of the stomach, while taking liquid, and also the changes in the nivean of the liquid in the stomach, by lifting the lower part of it, pressing with the hands, and the sinking down of it by ceasing to press.

The points by which the line tracing the organ is formed were indicated by those who made the examination, when they could distinctly hear the change in the sound, which was produced by passing the finger with some pressure over the skin.

CHAPTER III.

DIRECTIONS FOR OUTLINING THE VARIOUS ORGANS.

ANTERIOR PORTION OF THE BODY.

THE LUNGS.

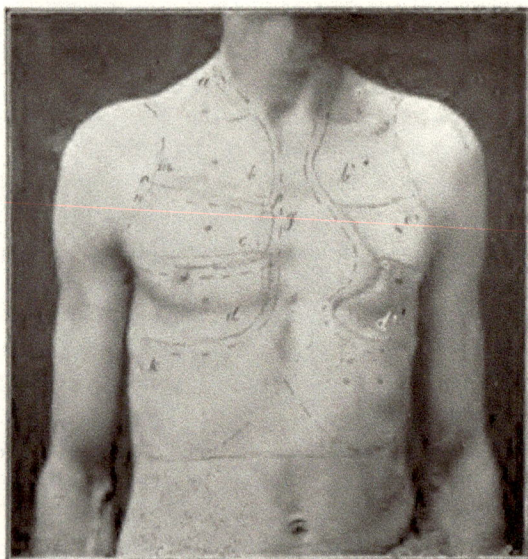

PHONENLOSCOPIC FIGURE OF LUNGS.

Place the Phonendoscope above, upon, and below the clavicle for the upper lobes (1–2); in the third intercostal space for the (4) middle lobe; in the fourth for the lower (5). *Do not stroke too hard.* In this way you can readily distinguish the beginning of the lung, its divisions into lobes, and the overlapping of the same. When a pleuritic effusion is present, put the instruments in the same positions, and, after examining in the upright and reclining positions, place the patient first on the right and then on the left side, to ascertain the variation in the level of the fluid. *Stroke vigorously.*

THE HEART.

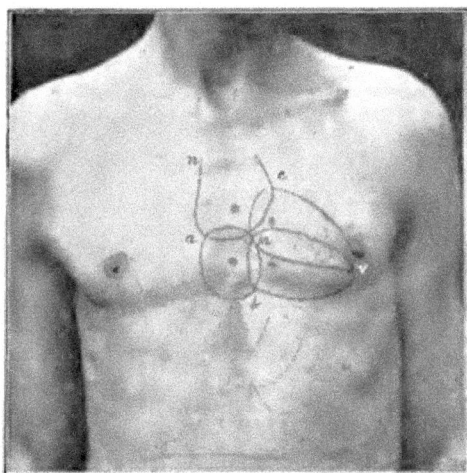

PHONENDOSCOPIC FIGURE OF HEART.

To determine the position of the heart, place the Phonendoscope in the left parasternal line, fourth intercostal space; for the right ventricle, a little lower to the left; for the right auricle, a little lower to the right; for the left ventricle, a little higher to the left; for the large vessels, a little higher to the right (arch of aorta, etc.); *vigorous strokes*. In this way we can determine the exact size and boundaries of the heart, its division into ventricles and auricles, and the position of the large vessels.

THE LUNGS AND HEART.

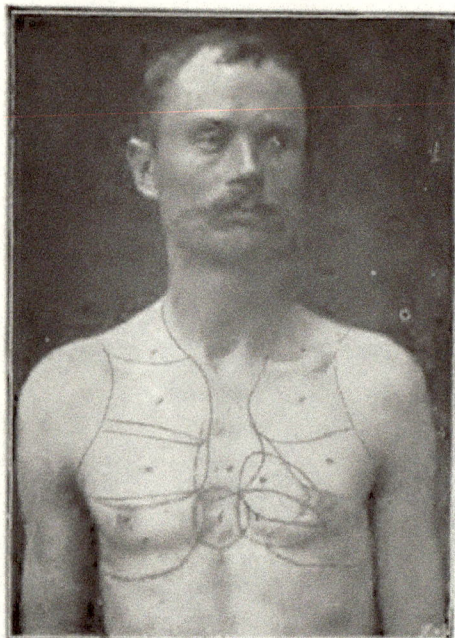

PHONENDOSCOPIC FIGURE OF LUNGS AND HEART.

THE LIVER AND COLON.

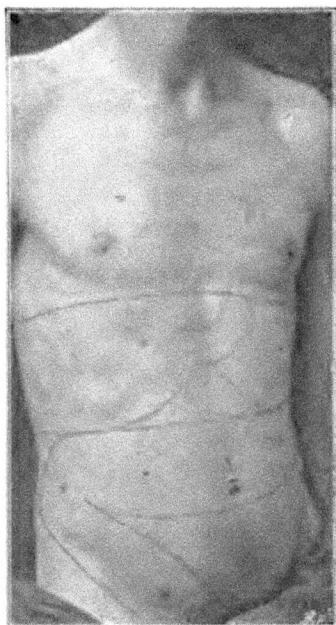

PHONENDOSCOPIC FIGURE OF LIVER
AND COLON.

THE LIVER.—Place the Phonendoscope in the following positions successively : Beneath the xyphoid appendix in the right mamillary line, in the seventh intercostal space : in the ninth intercostal space over the midaxillary line. *Vigorous strokes.*

THE COLON.—For the cæcum and ascending colon place the Phonendoscope in the right iliac fossa, beneath the free border and in the anterior axillary and midaxillary lines. For the transverse colon, on two or three points, according to the breadth, above a line which passes from right to left over the umbilicus and strikes the left free border between the midaxillary and posterior axillary lines. For the descending colon, beneath the left free border in the midaxillary line and also near the anterior superior spine of the ileum. *Stroking varies with the nature of the contents.*

THE STOMACH AND COLON.

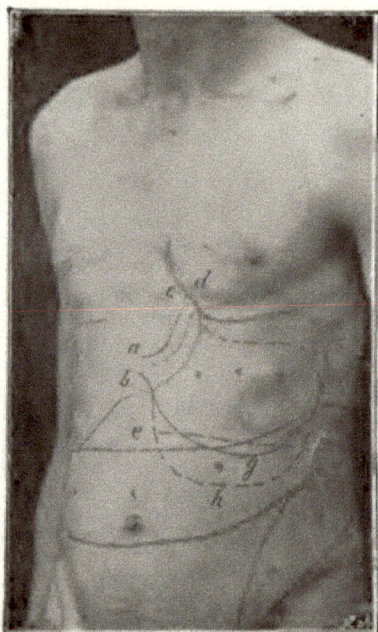

PHONENDOSCOPIC FIGURE OF STOMACH AND
COLON, WITH EXAMINATION POINTS.

THE STOMACH.—Place the Phonendoscope in the seventh intercostal space, left midclavicular line, and then on the linea alba near the left free edge of the ribs. When the stomach is full, place the instrument just below the greater curvature. We can thus distinguish the pylorus, cardia, the coils of the intestine, and the nature of their contents, whether fluid or gaseous, and also the change in place and form of the organs when the position of the patient is shifted. *Stroke vigorously for fluid, and lightly for gaseous contents.*

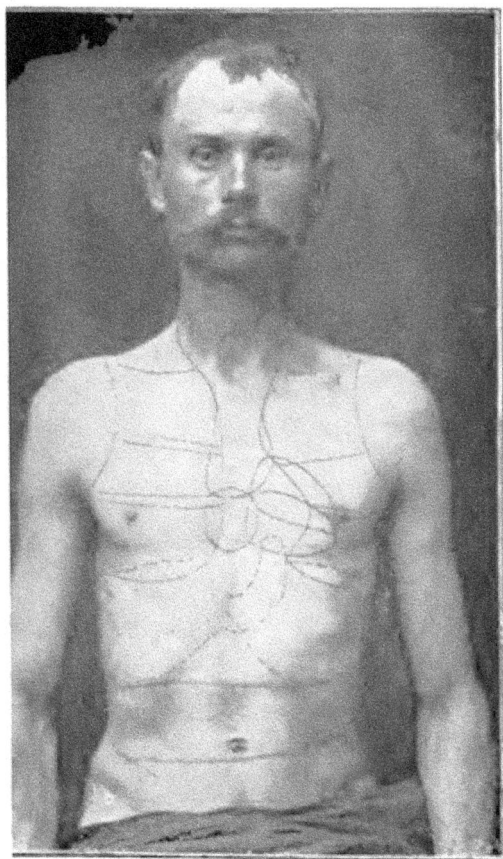

PHONENDOSCOPIC FIGURE OF FRONT SIDE OF BODY.

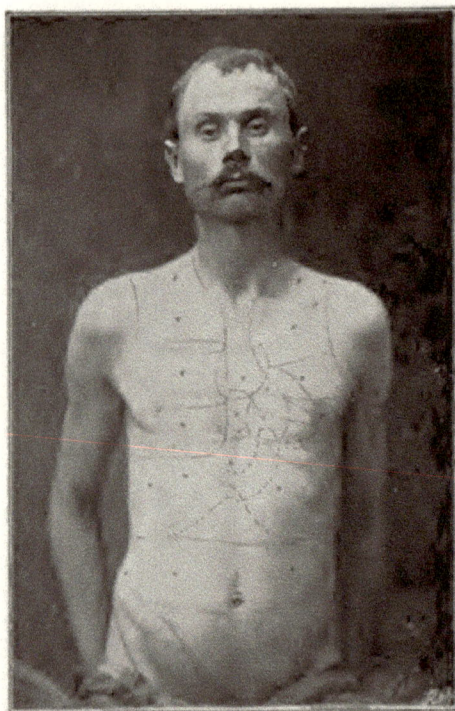

PHONENDOSCOPIC FIGURE OF FRONT SIDE OF
BODY, WITH EXAMINATION POINTS.

BLADDER.—Place the Phonendoscope in the linea alba above the symphysis pubis. *Stroke gently when the bladder is empty, vigorously when it is full of fluid.*

ASCITIC FLUID.—Place the Phonendoscope on either side in the anterior axillary line and in the linea alba on a level with the umbilicus, having the patient change from the upright to the reclining position, and even stand on his feet. *Stroke vigorously.*

NEW GROWTHS, *also deeply situated organs, as the kidneys and spleen,* can be outlined by placing the Phonendoscope over the centre of the organ and stroking the overlying region. *Enlarged glands* can be studied in the same way.

POSTERIOR SURFACE OF BODY.

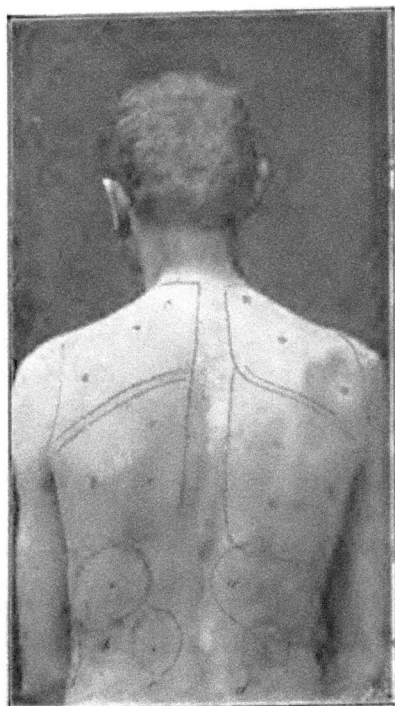

PHONENDOSCOPIC FIGURE OF BACK SIDE OF
BODY, WITH EXAMINATION POINTS.

LUNGS.—Place the Phonendoscope on either side in the scapular line at a level between the first and fourth dorsal vertebræ for the upper lobes, and between the seventh and tenth for the lower lobes.

LIVER.—Place the Phonendoscope in the right scapular region at the level of the twelfth dorsal vertebræ.

SPLEEN.—Place the Phonendoscope on the left side in the posterior axillary and midaxillary lines and in the interspaces between the last ribs.

KIDNEYS.—Place the instrument just within the semi-scapular line, immediately below the regions of the liver and the spleen.

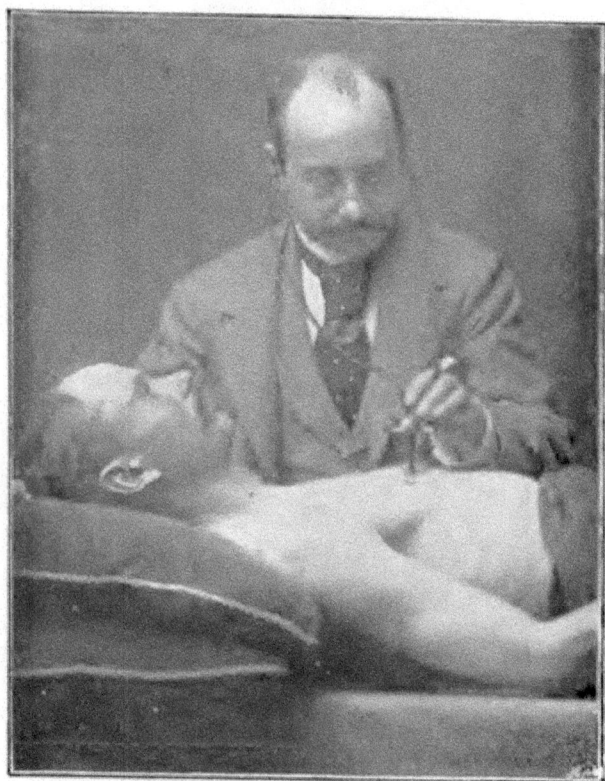

PHONENDOSCOPY OF NATURAL VIBRATIONS.

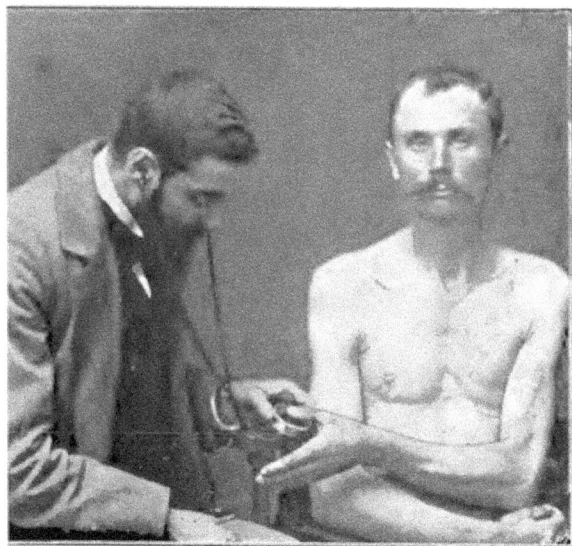

PHONENDOSCOPY OF MUSCULAR SOUNDS.

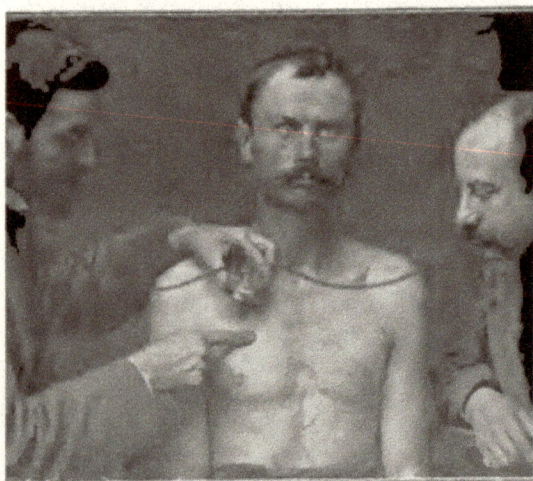

PHONENDOSCOPY OF VIBRATIONS ARTIFICIALLY PRODUCED.

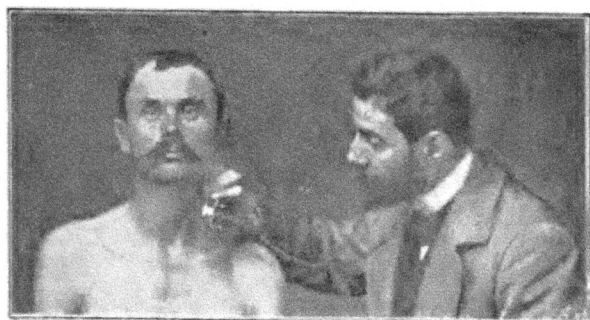

PHONENDOSCOPY OF LARYNX.

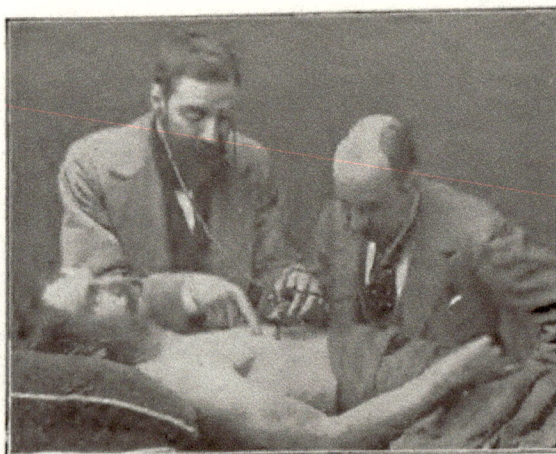

PHONENDOSCOPY OF VIBRATIONS ARTIFICIALLY PRODUCED.

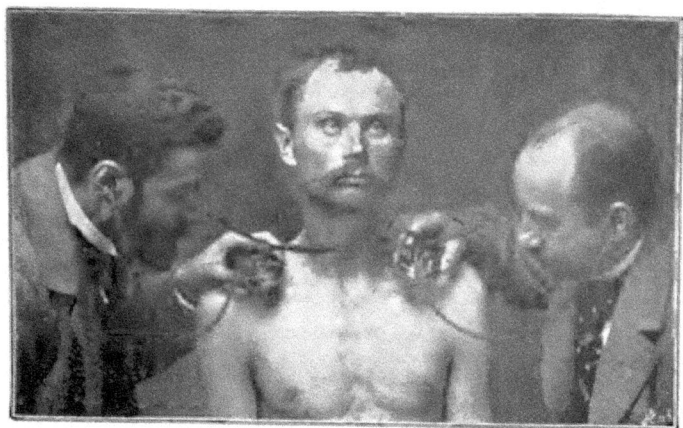

COMPARATIVE PHONENDOSCOPY.

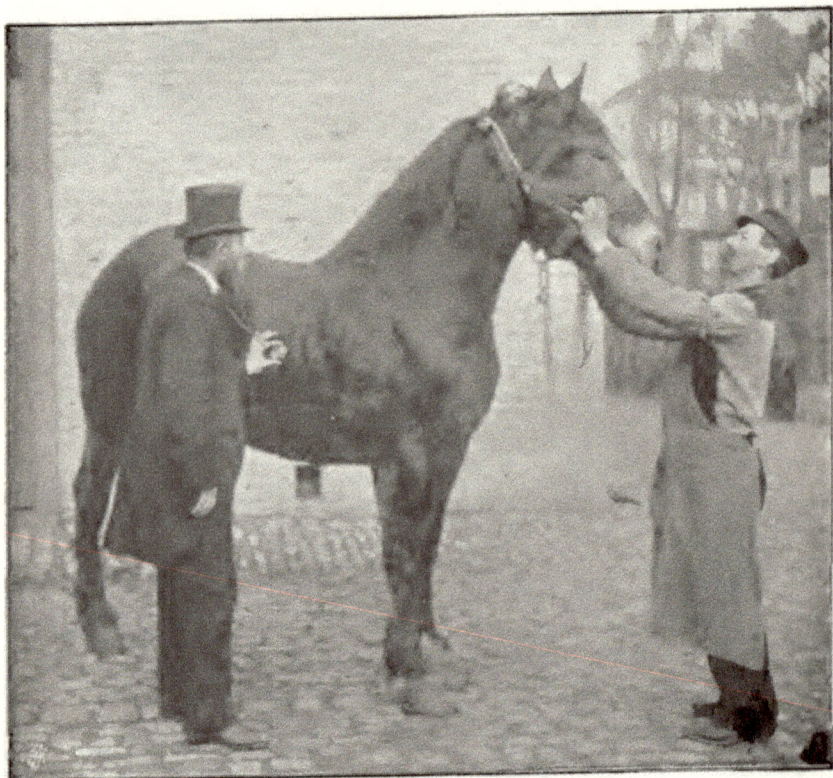

PHONENDOSCOPIC EXAMINATION OF HORSE.

FORKED ATTACHMENTS FOR THE PHONENDOSCOPE.

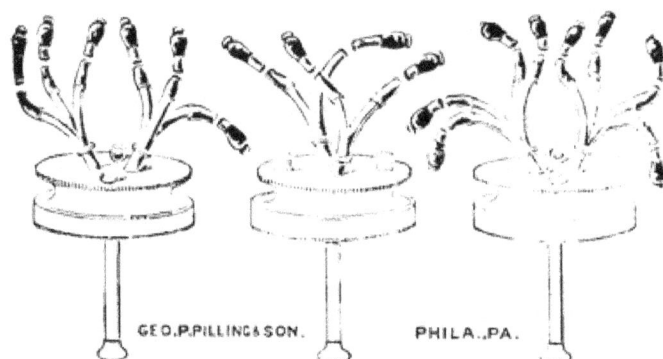

GEO.P.PILLING&SON.   PHILA.,PA.

The instances in which the Phonendoscope may be used simultaneously by a number of physicians are too numerous to mention. It very often happens that physicians when in consultation want to examine the same patient at the same time. If the physician only uses one ear then the regular tubes that come with the Phonendoscope will suffice, but if both the ears of each examiner are to be used then of course four tubes are required. For this purpose we have a set of tubes as shown in the center of the illustration in which it will be noticed that four tubes are attached. This simply is a Y-shaped fork. Thereby two or four physicians are enabled to examine with the same Phonendoscope. The figure on the left shows a triple fork, by means of which, either three or six physicians may examine at once with the same Phonendoscope. The other illustration shows a four-forked instrument with which four or eight physicians can examine at the same time with the one Phonendoscope. These attachments are very extensively used in the European Universities, especially during lectures, and when students are being instructed. These instruments were all made by George P. Pilling & Son, Philadelphia, and are most satisfactory, being made precisely like the samples obtained from Europe.

CHAPTER IV

THE RELATION BETWEEN THE OUTLINES OF THE INTERNAL ORGANS OF THE BODY AS DETERMINED BY THE X-RAYS AND BY THE PHONENDOSCOPE. THE LAWS GOVERNING THE TWO METHODS.

Those organs whose molecular vibrations in the form of light or sound make no sensible impression upon our sight or hearing without the use of specially constructed apparatus, are at the present time directly appreciable to the eye and the ear, on the one hand by the aid of the X-rays and Fluoroscope, and on the other by the aid of the Phonendoscope.

Skiascopy, therefore, the science of the X-rays and the Fluoroscope, and phonendoscopy, the science of auscultation with the aid of the Phonendoscope, are two new and far-reaching methods of studying the condition of the internal organs of the body both in health and disease; but these methods are still in their infancy.

Neither the vibrations of the cathode rays nor the sound-waves produced in the various organs of the body are appreciable to the eye or the ear, unless the eye be aided by the Fluoroscope, and the ear by the Phonendoscope.

While, on the one hand, the invisible vibrations of the X-rays penetrate the different viscera of the body with a facility which varies with the shape, density and mutual relations of the latter, and are then made visible in the Fluoroscope, or are fixed upon a photographic plate, so on the other hand, the friction of the finger-tip across the surface of the body gives rise to vibrations which are inaudible to the most acute ear, but which are taken up and intensified by the Phonendoscope, and so rendered distinctly audible. In this way the Phonendoscope outline of any desired organ may be traced upon the surface of the body.

Skiascopy and phonendoscopy are therefore two new clinical procedures, which give like results by different methods, the one rendering vibrations sensible to the eye, the other to the ear. Both methods may be made to give permanent results, the former by means of the X-ray photographs, the latter by means of the phonendoscopic chart.

The similarity of these results has led me to look for some constant relation between the two procedures in the hope of coming to some useful and definite conclusions. My efforts were rewarded with the most satisfactory results, and I can say without hesitation that both methods of procedure are governed by the same fundamental laws, and although each has its own peculiarities and variations the results of both are the same.

It was this consideration of the similarity of two methods of investigation so apparently different, one of which was discovered in Germany, the other in Italy, which has afforded me the opportunity of addressing this assembly to-day. I therefore beg to express my thanks to you for the honor of being present among you, and of being permitted to learn of progress, of new discoveries, of the fruits of investigation and experiment from the lips of the most prominent physicians of the German Empire.

You are well acquainted with the apparatus necessary for skiascopy; permit me to describe the instruments used in phonendoscopy. They are very few, consisting in fact of but one instrument, the Phonendoscope. The tip of the finger is used to stroke the skin for the production of the necessary vibrations, and an ordinary lead pencil suffices to draw the outlines of the organs upon the skin.

The Phonendoscope was invented at my suggestion about four years ago, and is the work of my colleague, Professor Bazzi. Since that time many imitations and modifications of the instrument have been made; these are, however, mere variations in the shape of the instrument and not in the principle of its construction.

With the aid of the Phonendoscope we can examine a large or a small portion of the body-surface with little difference in its sensitiveness. In fact it is just this power, afforded us by the use of the localizer, of examining one very minute portion of the body at a time, which has enabled me to develop a method of investigation which was never dreamed of before.

On account of the extreme sensitiveness of the instrument I have ceased using the forcible vibrations produced by the voice or by percussion, and have learned to utilize instead the very delicate vibrations produced by a gentle stroke of the finger across the skin.

The instrument is manufactured in Germany in the city of Cassel by the firm of Martin Wallach. This house not only manufactures a perfect instrument but spares no pains to distribute the same to all parts of the world.*

We now come to the subject proper of our paper.

(1) Neither skiascopy nor phonendoscopy cause the patient any pain.

(2) Neither the passage of the cathode ray through the body nor the scraping of the finger by which the vibrations for the Phonendoscope are produced cause the patient any pain, although the former occasionally gives rise to a burning or crawling sensation, in the skin the latter to an occasional tickling sensation.

(3) Neither the Fluoroscope, the sensitive photographic plate for the X-ray picture, nor the localizer of the Phonendoscope give rise to any other sensation to the patient than that of mere touch. The eye of the observer is apt to become tired after a prolonged examination with the Fluoroscope, as is also the ear of the physician using the Phonendoscope; but in the latter case the exhaustion is by no means as marked as in the former.

(4) In order to make the X-ray shadow in the Fluoroscope clear and distinct the instrument must be applied to the body at the point at which the organ to be examined is most superficial. In like manner the Phonendoscope must be applied to the surface directly over the desired organ, so as to bring it as far as possible into continuous contact with the organ itself.

(5) As the intensity of the X-rays must be adjusted according to the distance of the organ from the surface of the body, so it is also important to regulate both the pressure

---

*American agents are George P. Pilling & Son, Philadelphia.

exerted upon the localizer of the Phonendoscope and the force of the strokes by which the necessary vibrations are produced, according to the position of the organ to be examined. Very powerful X-rays will pass through the superficial and less dense structures of the body without producing a shadow; in using the Phonendoscope, if too much force be used in stroking the skin the pressure of the finger will increase the tension of the superficial structures and the vibrations will be transmitted to the deeper organs; and if too much pressure be made upon the Phonendoscope, the superficial vibrations will be suppressed and only those coming from the deeper organs will be transmitted through the instrument.

(6) In using the X-rays it is best to place the bulb opposite the viscus to be examined and the Fluoroscope directly over it, or if the viscus be a large one the Fluoroscope must be placed upon several different parts of its surface. In using the Phonendoscope, it should likewise be placed directly over the organ at one or more points according to the size of the organ, and the finger producing the vibration should move in a circular manner about the point of contact of the Phonendoscope with the body.

(7) With both the X-rays and the Phonendoscope we may obtain either a temporary result or a permanent record.

(8) In the case of the X-rays we may be satisfied with a simple examination of the viscera with the Fluoroscope with merely outlining the organs upon the skin.

(9) A permanent record can be obtained with either procedure by means of a photographic plate or a camera; but a phonendoscopic chart can be rapidly made if the outlines be drawn upon the skin with copying ink and a copy be made directly upon a sheet of paper.

(10) In order to obtain clear and trustworthy results with either the X-rays or the Phonendoscope, a thorough knowledge of the processes involved, an impartial judgment and technical skill are presupposed requirements.

(11) The outline obtained by either of these two procedures is not an exact representation of the outline of the viscus itself; it represents, rather, in one case the shadow of the viscus

upon the Fluoroscope, in the other the projection of the viscus
upon the surface of the body.   The farther a viscus is removed
from the surface of the body the more will its representation
be modified in various ways.   The position of the Fluoroscope
influences the shape of the shadow.   If the Fluoroscope is in
contact with one part of the body surface, for instance, the
anterior surface, the sides of the body and parts of organs
situated within the sides will be separated from the Fluoroscope
by some distance, owing to the oval contour of the body ;
hence arises a certain amount of distortion of the outline, or a
partial or general increase of its size.   In the case of the
Phonendoscope also, the fact that it can be brought to bear
upon the superficial surface of the organ only, and not even in
actual contact with that, and the fact that the body surface is
rounded cause the outline to assume a shape which is not the
actual shape of the organ itself.

(12)   The solid viscera throw a dark shadow upon the
Fluoroscope, whose intensity depends upon the density and
thickness of the viscus.   With the Phonendoscope it is found
that these same viscera give powerful vibrations whose intensity is directly proportionate to the thickness and density of
the viscera.

(13)   The shadow thrown upon the Fluoroscope by a solid
viscus situated in the posterior part of the body is darker in
the center of the shadow and lighter around its margin.   With
the Phonendoscope it is found that this same viscus gives rise
to vibrations which are more powerful at the center, where the
viscus touches the body wall, while towards its borders, where
the viscus is separated from the body wall, the vibrations
become less and less intense.

(14)   Viscera, consisting of one or more cavities containing gas give a brighter projection upon the Fluoroscope if the
tension of the gas is great ; and the greater the pressure of gas
in the viscera, the higher will be the pitch of the vibrations in
the Phonendoscope.

(15)   In a hollow viscus containing both gas and fluid,
the part containing gas will throw a light shadow upon the
Fluoroscope, the part containing fluid, a dark shadow.   In using
the Phonendoscope the part containing gas can be distinguished

from that containing fluid by the fact that the pitch of the vibrations over the gas is higher than over the fluid.

(16) Osseous structures throw a very dark shadow upon the Fluoroscope, and their vibrations in the Phonendoscope are high pitched. The shadows which any part of the body containing bone throws upon the Fluoroscope consists of the shadow of the bone plus the shadow of any organs lying behind the bone ; the tone of the vibrations heard in the Phonendoscope over a long part is a result of the blending of the vibrations peculiar to the bone with the vibrations from the underlying structures. The shadow thrown upon the Fluoroscope by an organ enclosed in a bony cavity is almost entirely obscured by the darker shadow of the bone ; in like manner the Phonendoscope is unable to detect the vibrations due to such organs on account of the predominance of the more powerful bony vibrations.

(17) The movements of the various viscera, whether physiologically or artificially produced, can be distinctly seen in the Fluoroscope by the motion of their shadows, provided, of course, that the X-ray bulb and the Fluoroscope remain stationary. In the case of the Phonendoscope, if the point of origin of the vibrations and the situation of the instrument are fixed, any change in the position of the underlying viscera can be determined by a change in their outlines as traced upon the skin. But such movements can be seen in the Fluoroscope in a limited number of organs only, such as the bones, the diaphragm, the heart and the lungs, whereas the Phonendoscope can be used on any part of the body and upon any viscus or part of a viscus, and upon accumulations of fluid in the different cavities of the body.

(18) If a viscus of a certain thickness and density lie directly behind another of the same density, their shadows will be superimposed upon the Fluoroscope and the result will be a single dark shadow ;—on the other hand, with the Phonendoscope we are able to differentiate such viscera and to outline them separately upon the surface of the body with as much facility as if they were transparent. This is accomplished by examining the superficial viscus first and then the deeper one. It is important in this case to apply the Phonendoscope at a

place where the superficial viscus comes into direct contact
with the body wall.

(19) A solid viscus or a viscus filled with fluid, situated
behind a hollow viscus, will throw a lighter shadow upon the
Fluoroscope in proportion to the thickness of the hollow viscus.
In using the Phonendoscope the vibration of the solid viscus
will likewise be found weaker, the greater the thickness of the
intervening layer of air.

(20) If the wall of a hollow viscus be thickened at any
point the shadow of the viscus will be less intense at the thickened point, for at this point the layer of air will be less deep or
even absent altogether. In the Phonendoscope the vibrations
over the thickened area will be much more powerful than over
the rest of the organ.

(21) Finally, by using two Roentgen bulbs and two
Fluoroscopes, corresponding organs of two individuals can be
examined and compared at the same time. In like manner,
two observers using two Phonendoscopes, can examine simultaneously and compare the vibrations of corresponding parts of
two subjects.

From the foregoing it will be seen that these two procedures are not only closely related, but are even somewhat similar; yet the use of the Phonendoscope has certain practical
advantages which are of special importance to the practicing
physician and which are not to be found in the present method
of using the X-rays. These advantages are to be found partly
in the nature of the apparatus and partly in the clinical application of the instrument.

The instruments required for phonendoscopy are very few.
The compact little instrument itself, a lead-pencil, some copy-
ing-ink and tracing paper to make copies of the phonendoscopic
chart. The tip of the finger produces the necessary vibrations.
The apparatus is portable, and can be used at any time and
place.

Clinically, we have already obtained results with the Phonendoscope which could not be obtained with the X-rays.

Not only are we able to trace with the Phonendoscope the
outlines of all the viscera, whether they are situated near the
surface or deep in the interior of the body, whether they are

solid or hollow or filled with gas or fluid, or even if they are suspended in the interior of a fluid cavity, but it also enables us to locate the subdivisions and ligaments of viscera, to determine all kinds of movements of the organs of the body or alterations of their positions as caused by their functional activity or through the action of gravitation.

Even an incomplete summary of the peculiarities of the Phonendoscope, such as can be given at this time must impress both the practicing physician and the scientist with the fact that the instrument affords us a rapid, easy and harmless clinical procedure, by means of which a projection of all the viscera may be traced upon the surface of the body ; and that the instrument will become popular and indeed indispensable to those who have studied its use carefully.

The application of the X-rays constitutes a most perfect method of controlling the results of the Phonendoscope, and there is no doubt that the X-ray apparatus will be improved in the near future so as to render their application much easier and the results more complete.

We trust that Germany, the home of the X-rays will soon realize this hope, for no problem however complicated can long remain a riddle to German scientists who are ever mindful of the proverb of the Tuscan Academia del Cimento, "Provando e riprovando."

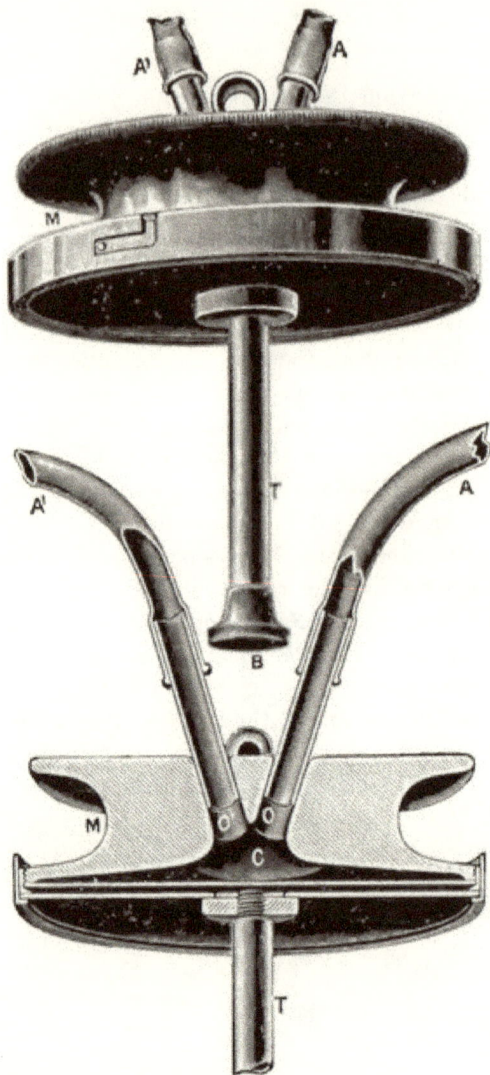

THE PHONENDOSCOPE.
NATURAL SIZE AND SECTIONAL VIEW.

CHAPTER V.

MECHANICAL DESCRIPTION OF THE PHONENDOSCOPE.

The Phonendoscope consists of the following parts: A solid metallic rod, T, terminating in a hard rubber bottom, B. This rod collects the vibrations and transmits them to a disc of hard rubber, sufficiently strong to withstand the pressure of the rod when it is applied to the body. This disc comes into contact with a second and thinner one of the same material, capable of vibrating easily. This thin disc is set into a mass of metal, M, of the size of a large watch. Between the disc and the mass there is an air space, C.

The interior thinner disc is more sensitive; the second stouter disc can easily be taken off, to uncover the interior disc. The sound produced by the disc is condensed by the metallic walls of this air space, and carried to the orifices, O and O', in which are fixed acoustic tubes, A and A'.

When examining the interior of an organ (such as the ear or the vagina), it is advisable to protect the small rod by a rubber tube, so that the sound is not conveyed away or weakened when the rod is touching the walls of the organ.

The ear tubes of India rubber have at one end an olivary ear-tip; the other end bears the metal tube to insert into the holes of the instrument. If, instead of plain metal tubes, a kind of forked tubes with several ends, are used, a number of persons can at the same time, and with one instrument, listen to the sounds made by the organ.

The object of this instrument is to render audible all sounds whether natural or caused by morbid conditions of the human body; they can be heard with much greater intensity and within much more narrow limits than it has been possible with the ordinary Stethoscope. At the same time it conveys with great accuracy the nature of the sound.

The Phonendoscope is useful for hearing :

(1) The sound of the respiratory organs, of the circulation of blood and of the digestive organs in the healthy body as well as in the sick subject.

(2) The sounds made by the muscles. joints and bones.

(3) The sounds in the matrix at the time of pregnancy and the noise provoked by the fœtus.

(4) The sound of the Capillary circulation.

(5) The slightest sound produced in any diseased condition of the body ; hence it is possible to draw on the body the dimensions, the position or any alteration in the position of the various organs and of the fluids which have gathered in the most important cavities of the body.

(6) The sounds in the ear, the eye, the bladder, the stomach, and the intestines.

The application of the Phonendoscope is quite easy ; it is placed with the outer disc on that part which is to be examined, and one or both the auricular tubes are placed to the ear or ears. In this way, both hands are free and the person examining the body can in the manner described below, determine the exact position and dimensions of an organ and mark its outlines on the body.

To get into practice with the Phonendoscope, it is recommended to listen at the beginning with one ear only and to institute a comparison between the direct auscultation and the examination made with the binaural Stethoscope. The superiority of the Phonendoscope compared with all other instruments will then be evident.

To examine extended parts of the body, the instrument is placed with outer disc on the part to be examined.

To examine limited parts (for instance, the sounds of the arteries and the heart), screw the small rod into the outer disc and press the rod cautiously and gradually against the part to be examined.

The various degrees of sensibility can be obtained in the following manner.

When applying the two discs and only one auricular tube, the instrument is the least sensitive.

By using the two auricular tubes and applying both discs, a medium degree of sensitiveness is obtained.

The highest degree of sensitiveness is obtained by removing the outer disc and applying only the interior disc and both auricular tubes.

Determining the outlines of the organs is not done by percussion, but by passing the forefinger with slight pressure over the organ in question, pressing during this manipulation the Phonendoscope with the small rod against the organ.

The following precautions are to be observed :

When examining the body, contact with clothes or other objects is to be avoided.

Press slightly and gradually with the instrument against the part to be examined, in order to secure a direct contact.

Avoid shocks or undue pressure on the interior disc.

Both auricular tubes are always to be inserted in the instrument, even when one tube only is required.

In comparison to the Stethoscopes the Phonendoscope offers the following advantages :

(1) Quick and reliable examination of one or several organs.

(2) Possibility of a summary, but exact examination, as well of dressed persons. In this case hold the instrument tight to avoid a rubbing at the clothes.

(3) Possibility of remaining distant from the patient, which is of considerable hygienical advantage to the physician and more convenient to the patient.

(4) Exclusion of disturbances through other noises in the examination room.

(5) Possibility of determining the outlines of the organs and drawing of same on the skin by marking the outlines with a colored pencil.

The Phonendoscope offers a certain method of detecting people who feign deafness. By placing the hard rubber tips in their ears, knocking gently on the rubber disc, let them tell in which ear they hear the noise, then press that tube with thumb and finger without patient's knowledge ; the sound is obstructed and simulation detected.

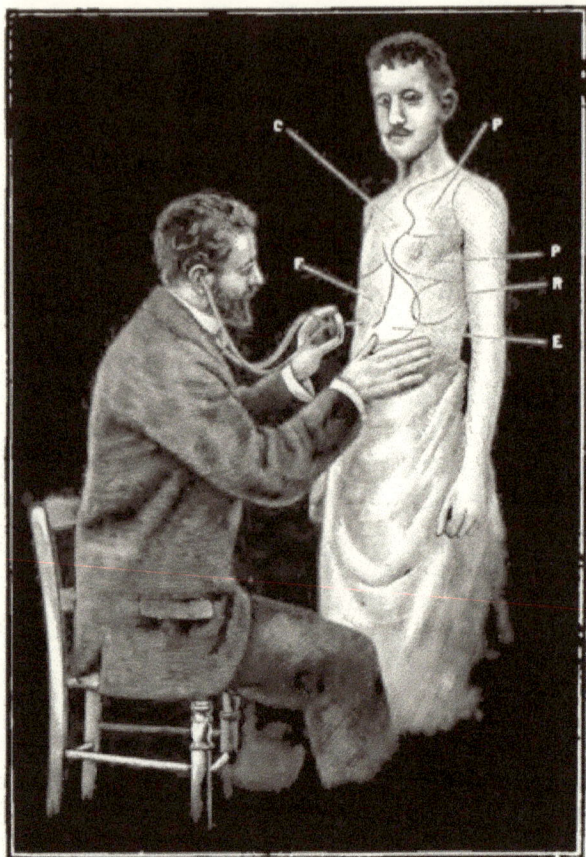

PROF. BIANCHI OBTAINING THE OUTLINES OF THE LIVER
BY MEANS OF THE PHONENDOSCOPE.

E, Stomach; F, Liver; C, Heart; P, P, Lobes of the left lung;
R, Spleen.

THE PHONENDOSCOPE AND THE DIGESTION OF FLUIDS.

By Felix Regnault, M. D., France.

The physician who would acquire a knowledge of the condition of the organs of the human body must use his ears for that purpose, in order that he may hear and understand the sounds produced, which are called into existence, whilst these organs, and internal parts of man, perform their various functions. But further than this: The physician, by means of percussion, may, himself, produce various sounds in these organs.

In order to do this, he places the middle finger of his left hand upon the spot, under which the organ which is to be examined lies concealed, and, with the finger-tip of his right hand, hammers or taps the middle finger of the left. By this procedure certain sounds are produced in the different organs: as, for instance, a solid organ, like the liver, or heart, or a bone, will give a heavy or dull sound. If the organ is light or empty, as the lungs and stomach, then the sound produced will be hollow and sonorous.

Now, in the course of disease, it may happen that an organ will give off a dull sound on percussion, which, when in its normal condition, would be sonorous. Thus it happens during the process of certain diseases of the lungs; as, in pneumonia and pleurisy, and other infiltrations, when the sounds of percussion will be dull. In a healthy condition, the clear resonance may be easily discerned, but this state changes with disease, and, therefore, it requires a well-trained ear to be able to distinguish the different sounds which may be produced, and thereby to ascertain the condition of any organ, so as to know whether it be diseased or enlarged or displaced.

It was the celebrated Dr. Piorry who excelled in making these distinctions. He had an instrument which he himself invented, and thus was enabled to discern the most subtle variations of sounds, and the condition of the organs. This instrument was the "Pleximeter." In the process of time Drs. Bianchi and Bazzi were anxious to simplify these methods of investigation.

In order to accomplish their purpose they constructed a new instrument, known as the Phonendoscope, and by its use the ear is enabled to ascertain the most minute differences in the sounds.

Now, the question arises, as to how the various sounds produced by percussion, which are scattered in every direction, and are thus carried away from the ear, which only receives a feeble part of the impulse of the sound-waves, could be carried directly, and in full, to the ear of the examiner? The answer is, that an instrument is needed for that purpose—an instrument, which receives the vibrations in full and conducts them, one and all, to our ears. The only instrument which will accomplish this purpose is the "Phonendoscope."

Now then, let us make an examination with this instrument. We will examine the heart. We select a given point upon the chest-wall with which the heart ought to be in direct contact on the inside. It is important that we make this selection, for, if a lobe of the lung should happen to intervene between the heart and the outer wall of the chest, then the instrument could not collect the sounds which are produced by the heart, as the greater part of them would be arrested by the lobe of the intervening lung. Now we place the button of the metallic rod upon the point selected, and we hold and press it perpendicularly against the thoracic wall, and thus depress the skin with the instrument. As the second finger of the right hand remains free, we use it to compress the skin, which is close to the organ we examine, and tap it with the point of this finger. Thus the organ which is situated beneath begins to vibrate, and these vibrations which the ear, unaided by any instrument, cannot perceive are transmitted to the Phonendoscope, where they become concentrated and intensified, and from which, by means of the acoustic tubes "A," "A," are accurately conveyed to the ears. And, as we remarked above, any intervening organ weakens the intensity of these sounds. It does not, however, obliterate them. Thus if a pulmonary lobe should intervene between the heart and the chest-wall, the finger striking it sets in vibration the heart, through the lung which intervenes.

We must remember that every organ, which is in immediate contact with the external pariets, will show its location above the skin, by an elevation, and thus, their form and contour may be outlined with a colored pencil.

The instrument invented by Dr. Bianchi, has still another advantage, which it shares with the Phonograph, and, that is, that many persons can listen at once by means of several tubes which may be attached to it, which is one of the greatest advantages in clinical instruction.

With the Phonendoscope you can hear the organs live and move, for, in fact, all our organs are in perpetual motion, and their positions only differ when different attitudes are assumed by the individual.

If we desire to obtain the most favorable results, we should examine phonendoscopically when our subject is standing upright.

The extent to which the organs are in contact with the pariets will be marked by a bulging out, or distention, over that particular area.

As an example marking the usefulness of recent discoveries, we have only to refer to the Phonendoscope.

We will now select the human stomach, as an example, on which we can try our skill, and realize the fruits of this discovery.

Heretofore every treatise on anatomy has selected the form of the stomach as found in the cadaver. You cannot outline it in this way upon a living subject. Percussion, especially, seems to be powerless, in recognizing the greater curvatures of this organ, when it is full of food. But by means of the Phonendoscope we recognize that the empty stomach is lengthened vertically more than anatomists have thought it to be, and when it receives food, it stretches itself still more in the same direction.

We will now drink a glass of water. Formerly, it was supposed that this water did not remain in the stomach. They said there was a special bundle of muscular fibers, called "La Cravate de Suisse," which by their contraction made the liquids pass directly from the cardiac to the pyloric end, *i. e.* from the oesophagus to the intestines. This whole view, which was once entertained, is absolutely erronious, as the "Cravate de Suisse" does not exist. The stomach retains liquids just the same as any other food. It empties itself as it rises, or draws itself up, as it were, lengthening or stretching itself transversely. The water level rises and reaches the pyloric orifice, and thus the fluids empty themselves by degrees, just as the lower curvature of the stomach rises.

Thus you will learn to appreciate the advantage of a dry diet for weak stomachs, because the liquid remains in it the same as any other food to be assimilated.

The weight imposed on this organ diminishes in proportion as we withhold fluids. Further, the stomach is taxed more or less, according to the nature and character of the fluids we drink. It is particularly interesting to study the variation of time in the digestion of different fluids in the human stomach. For this very reason we will be led to recommend to dyspeptics those liquids which are easily digested, and cause the smallest amount of trouble. We owe our thanks to Drs. Bianchi and Comte for the employment of the Phonendoscope, with which we can outline the empty stomach, when it is fasting, as given in figure "A." At the moment of the ingestion of one pint of fluid we have figure "B." And finally two hours after the ingestion we have figure "C."

These gentlemen have published the results of their experiments to the Medical Congress of Moscow, in a most remarkable report, of which we here affix an epitome for the benefit of the reader.

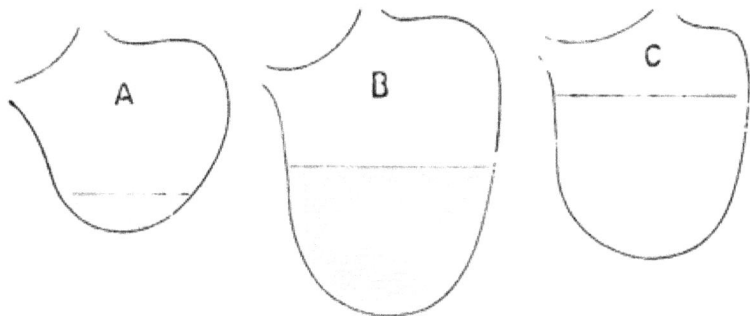

SELTZER WATER.

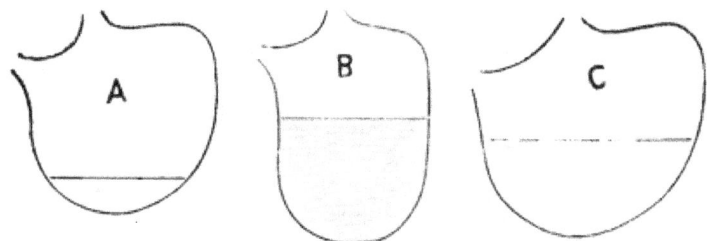

TEA.

WATER.

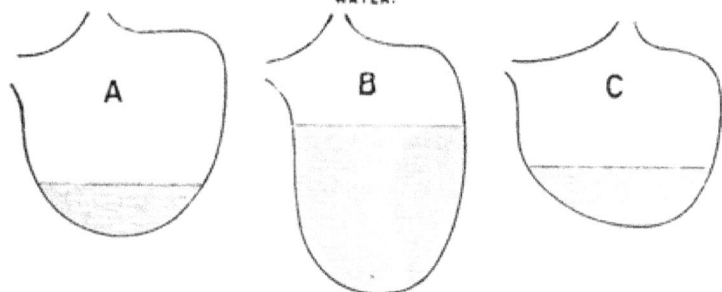

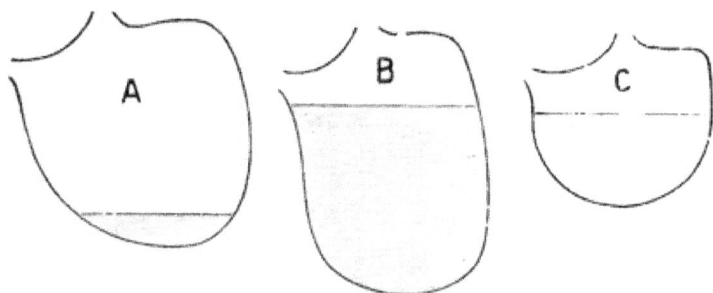

WINE.

DIGESTION OF WATER, WINE, SELTZER WATER AND TEA.

A, Stomach fasting; B, Form of stomach after the ingestion of two pints of liquid; C, Two hours afterward.

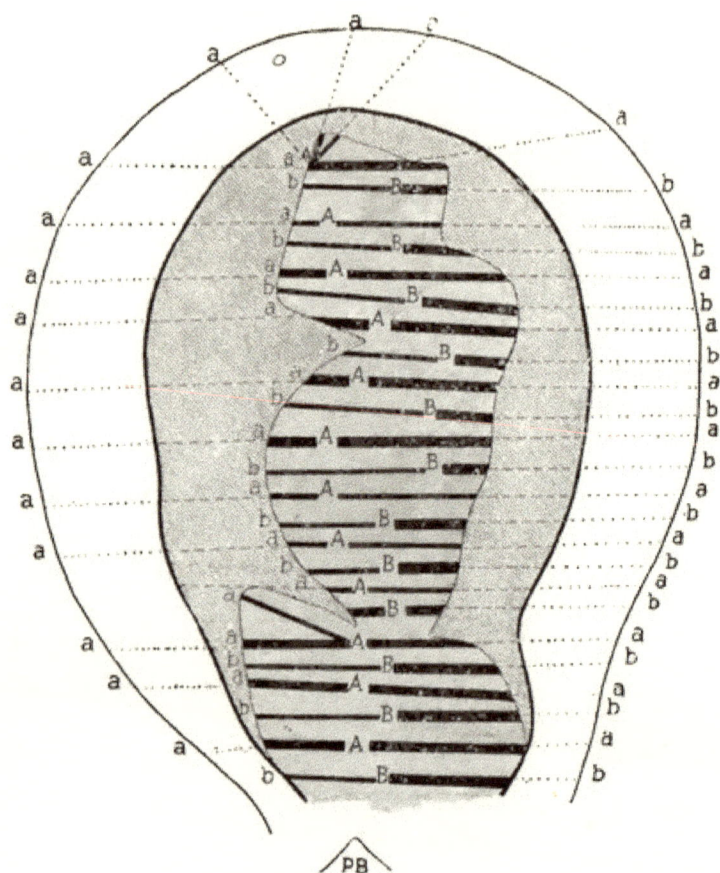

PHONENDOSCOPIC FIGURE 1.

A, Points of application for the stem of the Phonendoscope in the vicinity of the white line; B, Points of application on a lateral line for the fœtal location; P, B, Pubis; A, a, a and B, b, b, Lines indicating the proportions in the fall of the vibrations.

APPLICATION OF THE PHONENDOSCOPE IN THE COURSE OF PREGNANCY.

By Dr. M. Anastasiades, of Calamata, Greece.

The idea of using the instrument of Bazzi-Bianchi, as a means of investigation, suggested itself to us in the progress of a case of pregnancy. Our first attempt was made at the Charity Maternity Hospital, under the supervision of Professor M. Porack, to whom we owe our sincere thanks for the kind reception accorded to us.

After numerous experiments we are able to present to-day a certain number of observations which appear to us as the most convincing.

Our first efforts were made in the course of an advanced pregnancy, and were surrounded with difficulties, and discouraging in the beginning. However, after several trials, we were able to obtain results sufficiently conclusive, such as are presented in figure No. 3, which figure also represents our first complete phonendoscopic demonstration.

Before explaining our manner of procedure, we must say that the success of the examination depends upon the experience we may have in practicing phonendoscopy. We know that the stem of the Phonendoscope must be applied quite perpendicularly to the region which is to be examined, in order to receive the vibrations produced by the rubbings, according to their mode of undulating succession , as the sounds are propagated in the plates and the membranes in like manner. The organ beneath the skin enters into vibration by propagation, when it comes in contact with the same ; so that the ear perceived two groups of vibrations (those produced by the integment and the others by the organ to be explored) which make but one impression, being united into one sound. But when the most external organ ceases to vibrate, then the sound produced by the organ lying beneath this alone reaches the ear. This is an important point to be noted, because it helps us to determine the situation of the organ which lies beneath.

PHONENDOSCOPIC FIGURE 2.

A, Points of application of the stem of the Phonendoscope on the white line for the uterine marking (location). B, Points of application of the stem for the uterine location, as counter-proof. D, D, Great and little uterine donicity. P, B, Pubes.

It is absolutely necessary to know that when the skin is insufficiently distended, or when moist it is not favorable to phonendoscopic examination ; and, on the other hand, that exaggerated tension of the external parts induces vibrations that drown those of the organ beneath. It is therefore necessary that we apply the stem and practice the rubbings in a manner suited to the physical condition of the skin, varying according to the individual requirements, and, in the same individual. in the different regions, etc., etc.

It is also necessary to remember that the vibrations, produced in too close a proximity to the stem, when pressure. more or less strong, is applied, so as to put the skin in contact with the organ beneath, which is to be examined. are of no value whatever. We must also bear in mind the fact that the muscles enter into vibrating process, and give a sound which reaches the ear, with those of the wall, and of the organs beneath. It is necessary, therefore, to pay the greatest attention to that which happens on the surface, but we may say that the vertical rubbings, during the examination of the foetal regions, do not set the fibres in action. In general, skin which is stretched too much causes vibrations which drown those of the organs beneath, and skin too much relaxed gives no vibrations at all. Also to facilitate the examination we have in course of construction a complimentary appliance which will, we hope, overcome all these difficulties. As to the rubbings, they must be made with the point of the finger, always by successive tappings (palpations), going from the inside outward, very closely to the stem. It is necessary to make a sort of rubbing percussion, starting from the stem of the instrument, and in going away from it, following a horizontal line.

This is the sum total of these technical details which are acquired only by practice. Let us now pass to the examination of a pregnant uterus. The pregnant woman is laid flat on her back, the shoulders slightly raised, after emptying the bladder we apply the stem of the instrument to the white line, no matter at what point, to the umbilicus for example, and quite perpendicularly to the skin's surface, and pressing more or less, according to the depth of which we have judged approximately the uterus is to be found, and according to the

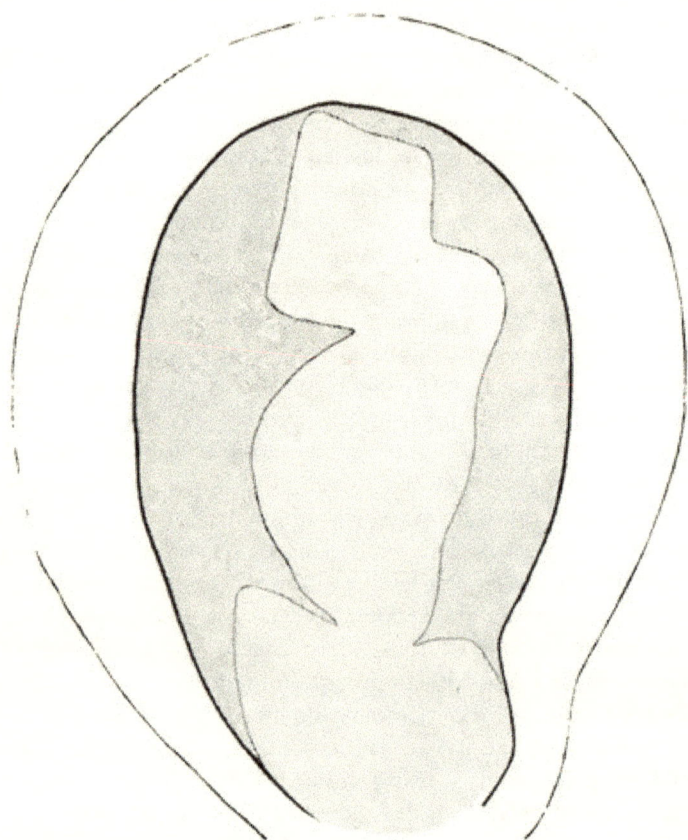

PHONENDOSCOPIC FIGURE 3.

Schema representing the great, the little donicity and the fœtus of a
pregnancy of eight months, left position.

thickness of the skin. We then begin the rubbings with the point of the finger, proceeding to make a succession of close, quick strokes, starting at the stem, and going away from it in a transverse line. When we arrive at a point where the sound diminishes, in a decided manner, we make a mark with a colored pencil, then repeat the same operation. following in the same horizontal line on the other side of the stem. After that we continue the rubbings further on from this point, and always following in the same line until the ear can no longer detect any sound, then we must mark this new point. We repeat the operation on a second horizontal line three centimeters from the vertical, above the preceding, and on the entire length of the white line above and below the umbilicus. To obtain the exact limits, and by way of control, we perform the same series of operations, following two vertical lines, each traced parallel by three or four centimeters to the right and left of the middle umbilical line. We thus obtain two series of marks. the ones corresponding to the points where the sound diminishes abruptly, and the others to those where it ceases altogether. We unite the marked points, and thus obtain two concentric curves or cycloforms, which present the figure of the uterus. giving in a way the outlines of a vertical curve, and following its anterior surface. The interior curve corresponds to the part of the uterus which is in contact with the abdominal wall, it is the little uterine echo chamber of the foetal sounds or vibrations. The large curve corresponds to the parts which run from the wall ; it is the great echo chamber of the same sounds.

The depth of the uterus answers to the mark which joins the extreme superior points : but for greater exactness we can outline neighboring organs. This we accomplish by making a series of rubbings directed from below upwards on the middle and lateral lines already traced. A little practice will enable us to make these various operations with great rapidity. In this manner we locate the uterus. Now how can we locate the foetus ? For locating the foetus we place the woman on her knees, near the edge of the bed, make her bend over, being supported by the shoulder of some one placed in front of her, or on any kind of support in such a way so that the body makes a sharp angle, in a horizontal attitude, so that the opera-

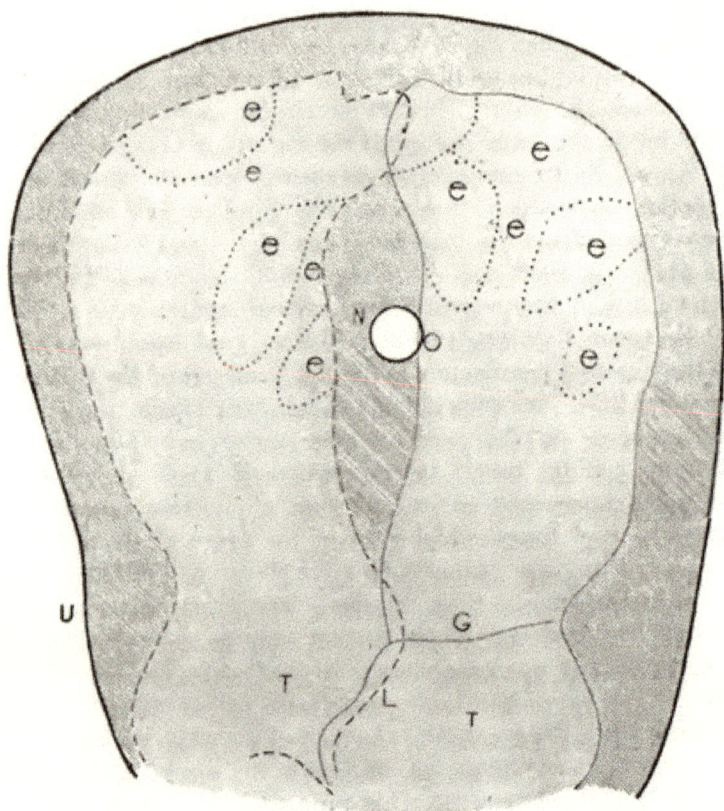

PHONENDOSCOPIC FIGURE 4.

Schema representing a gemillaire, or twin pregnancy of eight and a-half months, amniotic liquid in excess; U, Uterus; O, Umbilicus; N, Zone neutral; T, T Fœtal heads; G, Lines showing the head and body; e, e, e, Unsteady fœtal inferior extremities.

tor may be able to make his examination more freely. It is true that by this position the abdominal walls are more or less stretched, but we must try to modify this condition by changing the position of the subject now and then, so as to lessen the contractions. In this position the uterus swings and comes against the abdominal wall, except in its most inferior part. For the phonendoscopic research of the foetus, we take two lines chosen, after a preliminary palpation, which indicates the region of most resistance, lines which we follow, as for the determination of uterine sound limits. The stem of the instrument being placed we make the rubbings by going from the inside outward, long, vertical, and quite hard. Where the sound changes we mark a point ; then recommence the same operations as for the sound limits, the divers points thus obtained are compared to each other, and mark the foetal line.

For this foetal "schema" or figure it is to be noted that the kneeling position is the most favorable, because in this position, the foetus comes in contact with the anterior wall of the uterus, and by its own weight displaces the amniotic liquid. However, the inferior part of the uterus is kept away from the wall, and in order to explore it, it is necessary that the dorsal position be assumed, the seat being sufficiently elevated. This is done after having traced the schema or figure of the superior part, according to the first position. In the horizontal position only can we obtain, sometimes, the entire foetal schema or form ; thus it is that schema or figure No. 1 was obtained complete in these two positions. But we often meet with difficulties, when the foetus is very unsteady, or when the amniotic liquid is very abundant, as was the case in schema or figure No. 2, which we could not have obtained otherwise than in the kneeling position. (It is generally necessary to know how to combine the two positions.) We here produce three schemas which represent the same foetus. In one case, as you see, we have been able to diagnosticate a gemillaire or twin pregnancy. It would be very difficult for us to say just now what place this mode of obstetrical examination will hold in comparison with the palpation, soundings and other processes. However, it seems to us that the results already obtained are sufficient to say that phonendoscopy will be of real service, not only in the

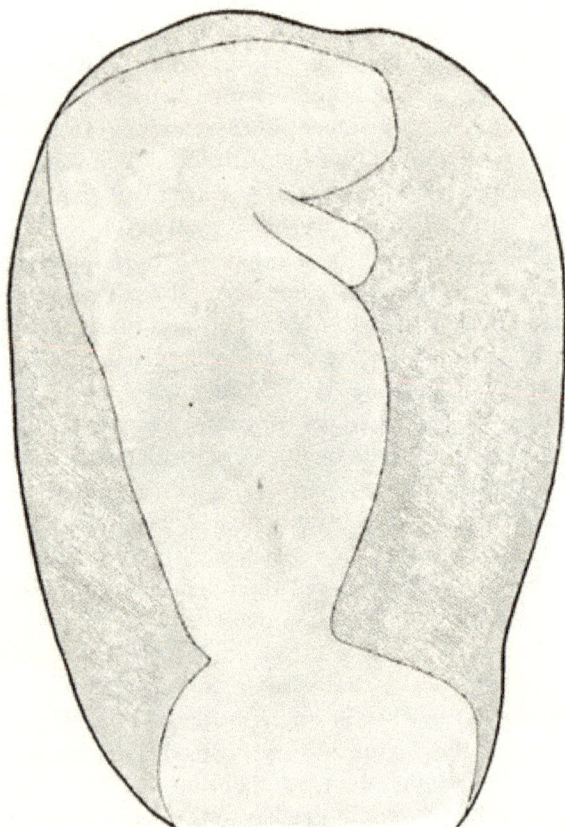

PHONENDOSCOPIC FIGURE 5.

Fœtal schema, right position, pregnancy complete,
abdominal wall very thick.

diagnosis of simple cases of pregnancy, *i. e.*, normal cases, but more especially in cases of hydrocephalus, and twin pregnancies, and of various anomalies of the uterus, etc., where the other modes of examination are very often without avail.

BAZZI=BIANCHI

Phonendoscope

Patented in U. S. A. and most of the civilized countries

Trade-Mark "PHONENDOSCOPE" registered in
U. S. Patent Office

GEORGE P. PILLING & SON

PHILADELPHIA

HECTOR T. FENTON, PHILADELPHIA
Patent Counsel

Sole Agents for the
U. S. A.

BEWARE OF IMITATIONS

All Genuine Instruments sold in U. S. A. stamped
with our name.

PRICES OF THE
PHONENDOSCOPE

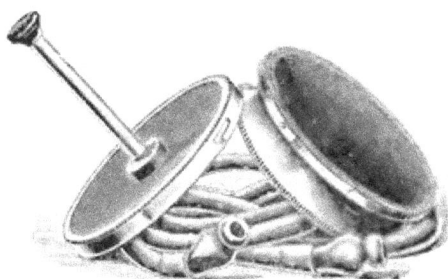

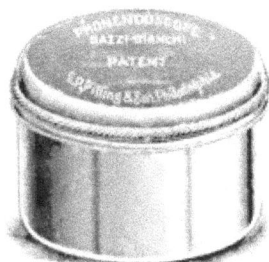

NO. 1 CASE. METAL, NICKEL PLATED

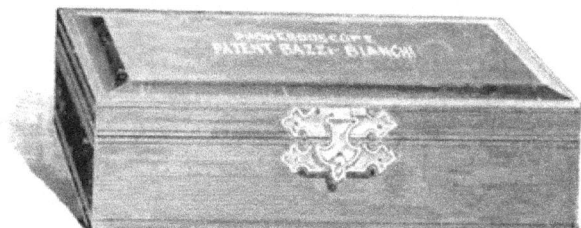

NO. 2 CASE. VELVET LINED

In No. 1 Case, $3.75   In No. 2 Case, $4.00

May be purchased from your surgical dealer, or, if not in stock,
from us direct.

GEORGE P. PILLING & SON

1225-27-29 Callowhill Street

PHILADELPHIA, U. S. A.

MARTIN WALLACH, Nachfolger, Cassel, Germany and Rome, Italy
European Agents for Phonendoscope

Phonendoscope

—CHILDREN'S SIZE

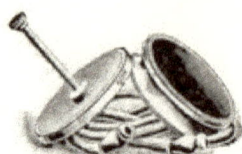

SOME time ago we were urgently requested to manufacture a smaller size of the Phonendoscope. We hesitated, not wishing to vary from the Bazzi-Bianchi standard, but finally made up a few, exactly same style and proportions as the standard but about three-quarters the size. We forwarded one of these to Martin Wallach, Nachfolger, and Prof. Aureli Bianchi. Both Wallach and Prof. Bianchi report very favorably and recommend it for children's use. We therefore designated this as the "CHILD'S SIZE" and it should be so stated when ordering. We do not want to complicate ordering, so please notice that in ordering the regular standard Phonendoscope it is not necessary to state size, AS THE STANDARD WILL ALWAYS BE SENT unless "Child's Size," is specified.

Prices of Child's Size, same as Standard

GEORGE P. PILLING & SON

Sole Agents for U. S. A.   PHILADELPHIA, PA.

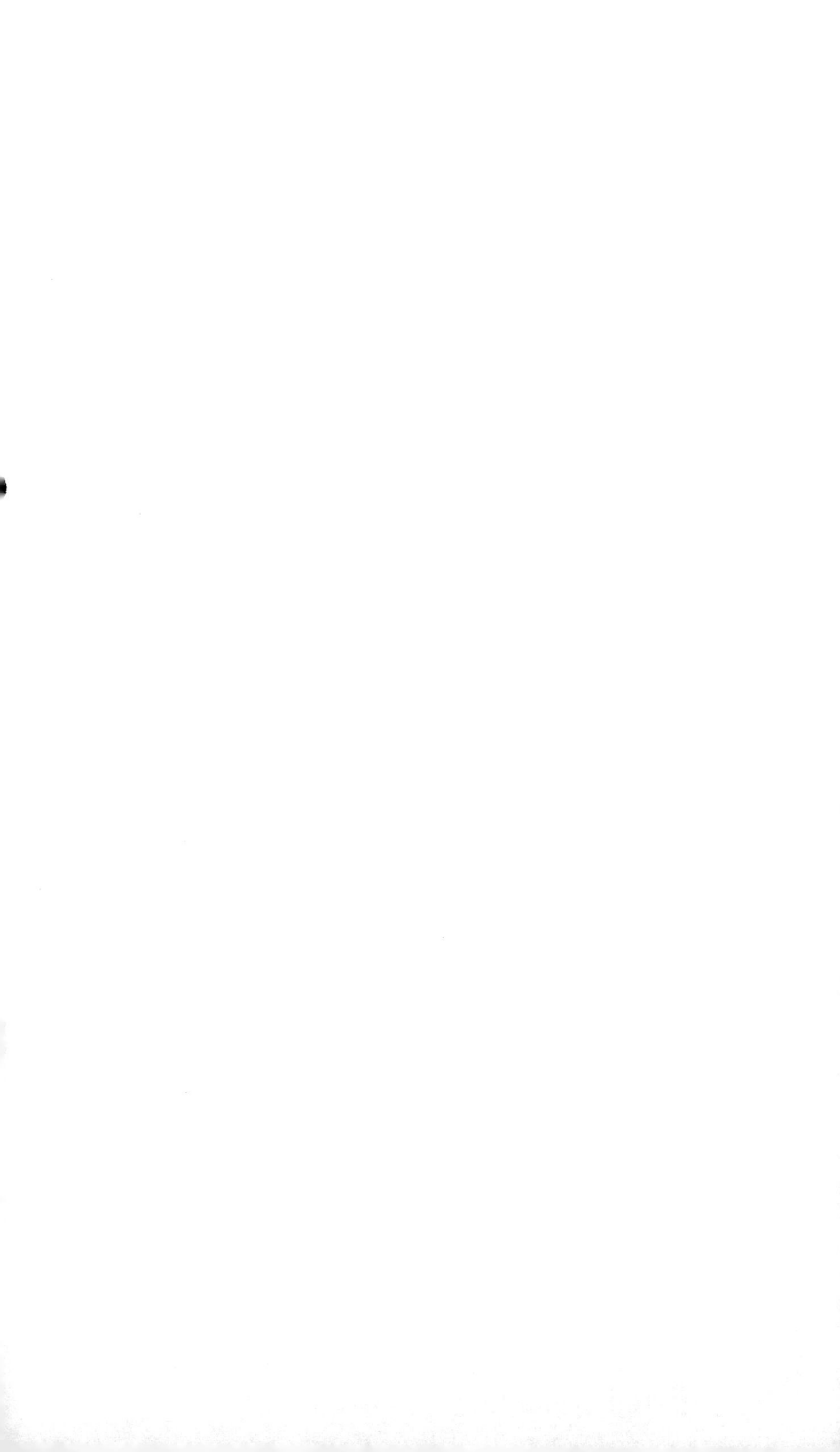